Living with a Person with Dementia

of related interest

What You Really Want to Know About Life with Dementia
Real stories and expert advice for family, friends and people with dementia
Karen Harrison Dening, Hilda Hayo, Christine Reddall
Foreword by Keith Oliver
ISBN 978 1 78775 695 3
eISBN 978 1 78775 696 0

The Family Experience of Dementia
A Reflective Workbook for Professionals
Jack Morris and Gary Morris
Foreword by Kate Swaffer
ISBN 978 1 78592 574 0
eISBN 978 1 78450 983 5

Dear Alzheimer's
A Diary of Living with Dementia
Keith Oliver
Forewords by Professor Linda Clare and Rachael Litherland
ISBN 978 1 78592 503 0
eISBN 978 1 78450 898 2

Dementia Support for Family and Friends, Second Edition
Dave Pulsford and Rachel Thompson
ISBN 978 1 78592 437 8
eISBN 978 1 78450 811 1

LIVING WITH A PERSON WITH DEMENTIA

An A–Z of Strategies for Successful Support

Bernie McCarthy

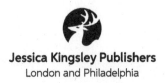

Jessica Kingsley Publishers
London and Philadelphia

First published in Great Britain in 2025 by Jessica Kingsley Publishers
An imprint of John Murray Press

1

Copyright © Bernie McCarthy 2025

The right of Bernie McCarthy to be identified as the Author
of the Work has been asserted by him in accordance with
the Copyright, Designs and Patents Act 1988.

Front cover image source: Nicola Powling. The cover image is for
illustrative purposes only, and any person featuring is a model.

All rights reserved. No part of this publication may be reproduced, stored
in a retrieval system, or transmitted, in any form or by any means without
the prior written permission of the publisher, nor be otherwise circulated
in any form of binding or cover other than that in which it is published and
without a similar condition being imposed on the subsequent purchaser.

The information contained in this book is not intended to replace the services
of trained medical professionals or to be a substitute for medical advice. You
are advised to consult a doctor on any matters relating to your health, and in
particular on any matters that may require diagnosis or medical attention.

A CIP catalogue record for this title is available from the
British Library and the Library of Congress

ISBN 978 1 83997 382 6
eISBN 978 1 83997 383 3

Printed and bound in Great Britain by Clays Ltd

Jessica Kingsley Publishers' policy is to use papers that are natural,
renewable and recyclable products and made from wood grown in
sustainable forests. The logging and manufacturing processes are expected
to conform to the environmental regulations of the country of origin.

Jessica Kingsley Publishers
Carmelite House
50 Victoria Embankment
London EC4Y 0DZ

www.jkp.com

John Murray Press
Part of Hodder & Stoughton Ltd
An Hachette Company

The authorised representative in the EEA is Hachette Ireland,
8 Castlecourt Centre, Dublin 15, D15 XTP3, Ireland (email: info@hbgi.ie)

Contents

Introduction   11

PART I: THE RELATIONSHIP COMPASS   13

Expert – I know (and you don't)	14	Needs	21
Columbo – You know (and I don't)	14	Physical environment	27
Collaborator – We both know	15	A word about the brain and dementia	27
Companion – Neither of us knows	15	Emotions	30
Moving from one position to another	16	Foundations – what behaviour is	33
Why do people with dementia do the things they do?	17	ABC model of behaviour	33
		Behaviour change	34
Physical health	18	Attachment, caregiving and dementia	35
Emotions	19	Responses and strategies to avoid	40
Personality	20	Behavioural approaches to use	45
Memories and trauma	20	Caring for yourself in it all	52

PART II: A–Z OF DEMENTIA CARE AT HOME   53

A

		Announcing care	63
Absconding	53	Annoyed	63
Abuse (in the past)	53	Antecedent	64
Abuse (in the present)	54	Anti-anxiety medication	64
Accusations	55	Antidepressant medication	64
Activity	56	Antipsychotic medication	65
Adynamia	57	Anxiety	65
Aggression	57	Apathy	67
Agitation	60	Art	67
Agnosia	61	Assault	68
Alcohol	62	Assertiveness	69
All-or-nothing thinking	62	Assisting	69
Alzheimer's disease	63	Attachment	70

Attention	70	**D**	
Attention-seeking	70	Dad	93
		Dance	94
B		Death	94
Back off	71	Decision-making	95
Bathing	72	Defences	96
Bedwetting	74	Defensiveness	96
Behaviour	74	Delusions	96
Behaviour Support Team	75	Delirium	97
Behavioural consequences	75	Dementia	98
Bereavement	76	Denial	99
Black-and-white thinking	77	Dentist	100
Boredom	77	Depression	100
Boundaries	78	Dignity	100
Brain	78	Disempowerment	101
Brain cells	79	Disparagement	101
Burnout	79	Disruption	102
		Distraction	102
C		Distress behaviour	102
Caregiving	80	Disturbed behaviour	103
Catastrophizing	81	Domestic tasks	103
Causes, behavioural	81	Double entendre	104
Celebration	81	Dressing	104
Challenging behaviour	81	Driving	105
Choices	82	Dying	106
Church	83		
Closeness	83	**E**	
Cognitive behavioural		Eating	106
therapy (CBT)	84	Emotions	107
Cognitive distortions	85	Empathy	109
Cognitive rehabilitation (CR)	85	Empowerment	110
Cognitive stimulation		End of life	110
therapy (CST)	85	Enjoyment	110
Collaboration	86	Ethics	111
Comfort	86	Excess disability	112
Communication	86	Executive function	112
Competence, legal	87	Exercise	113
Compliments, praise	88		
Confabulation	88	**F**	
Consent	88	Facilitation	113
Consequences	89	Faith	113
Continence	89	Family	114
Conversation	91	Fear of strangers	114
Cooperation	92	Fears	115
Coordination problems	92	Feeding	115
Creativity	92	Feelings	116
Cynicism	93	Financial planning	117
		Finger-food	117
		Fitness	119

Forgetting	119
Friends	120

G
Gardening	120
Gestures	121
Going out	121
Guardianship	122
Guilt	122

H
Hallucinations	123
Happiness	125
Health	125
Hearing	126
Helplessness	126
Hitting	127
Hobbies	128
Holding	128
Home	128
Hope	129
Housework	129
Hugging	129
Humour	130
Hunger	130
Hygiene	131

I
Identity	131
Ignoring	132
Ill-being	132
Illness	133
Implicit memory	133
Imposition	134
Inclusion	134
Incontinence	135
Independence	135
Indifference	135
Infantilization	136
Insomnia	136
Intact abilities	137
Intimacy	137
Intimidation	138
Invalidation	138

J
Jokes	138
Joy	138

L
Labelling	139
Language	139
Laughter	139
Learning	140
Leaving home	140
Lewy body disease (LBD)	140
Life story	141
Light	142
Likes/dislikes	142
Limit setting	143
Listening, active	143
Long-term memory	145
Love, affection	145
Lying	146

M
Malignant social psychology	147
Mealtimes	147
Medication	148
Memory	149
Mirroring	149
Mirrors	149
Mistakes	150
Misunderstood, being	150
Mobility, loss of	151
Mocking	151
Mother	151
Motivation for behaviour	151
Music	152

N
Nagging	153
Nakedness	153
Names	154
Needs	154
Negotiation	154
Noise	155
Non-verbal communication	156

O
Objectification	157
Obsessions	157
Occupation	158
Outbursts	158
Outpacing	159
Overeating	159

P

Pain	160
Palliative care	161
Parents	161
Passivity	163
Pauses in conversation	164
Perception	164
Personality	166
Person-centred care	167
Personhood	168
Photographs	169
Physical environment	169
Play	170
Positioning	171
Positive and Negative Signs Scale (PANSIS)	172
Positive person work	172
Post-traumatic stress disorder (PTSD)	172
Power battles	174
Privacy	174
Problem behaviour	175
Psychological therapies	175
Psychosis	176
Punishment	176
Purpose, sense of	177

Q

Quality of life	177

R

Reaching through dementia	178
Reactions to behaviour	178
Reading	178
Reality orientation	179
Recall memory	180
Recognition memory	180
Recognizing faces	180
Recreation	180
Refusal	181
Regression	181
Reinforcement	181
Relationships	182
Relatives	182
Religion	182
Reminiscence	183
Repair	183
Repetitiveness	183
Repression	184

Reprimand	185
Respite	185
Routine, daily	186

S

Sadness	187
Safeguarding	187
Scaffolding	187
Scolding	187
Screaming	188
Sedation	188
Self	189
Self-esteem	189
Self-harm	190
Sex	190
Sexual assault	191
Sexual disinhibition	192
Shopping	192
Short-term memory	193
Shouting	194
Sleep	194
Smell	195
Smiling	195
Socializing	195
Soiling	196
Spirituality	196
Spitting	197
Stigma	197
Stimulation	197
Stress	197
Suffering	198
Sundowning	199
Surviving as a carer – Tom Valenta's Ten Golden Hints (Valenta, 2007)	200
Swearing	200

T

Talking books and podcasts	201
Taste	201
Teamwork	202
Tears	202
Teeth	202
Telling lies	203
Temperature	204
Time-out for you	204
Tiredness	204
Toilet	205
Tone of voice	206

Touch	206	**W**		
Trauma	206	Wandering	213
Treachery	207	War	214
Trust	208	Way-finding	214
		Well-being	215
U		Will	215
Unsafe leaving	208	Withdrawal	215
Urinary tract infections (UTIs)	209	Work	215
		Worship	216
V		Writing	216
Validation	210		
Vascular dementia	211	**Y**	
VIPS	211	Yelling	216
Vision	212	Younger onset dementia	216
Visiting	213		
Vocabulary	213		

Appendix 218

References 220

List of Topics 221

Introduction

If you are reading this book, I assume it is because you have some contact with a person with dementia or a reason for wanting to know more about how to relate with a person with dementia. Or you may have had difficulties that you want some help with.

Dementia care is a partnership between two or more people with different roles. This book is written for the people in the partnership who do not have dementia. They may have their own forgetfulness and other problems that make life difficult. However, their role is to provide support to those with a diagnosis of dementia.

The role of living with and caring for a person with dementia is akin to being a Sherpa for a mountaineer who requires the guidance and support of your knowledge and skills to climb the mountain of dementia.

> Sherpa originally referred to the tribe in Nepal whose social custom was to provide humane and courageous mountain guides to outsiders. (Urban Dictionary)

You know the peaks and valleys of their lives, their personalities, their life stories and can respond to their need, moment to moment. You help them without doing it for them. You do not take over but support them so that the person with dementia can succeed. Sometimes this requires very little support and on other occasions it requires the sensitivity to judge the moment and provide just the right amount and type of support at just the right time.

Sherpa is an honourable role and attracts great respect. It is not

LIVING WITH A PERSON WITH DEMENTIA

possible for strangers to ascend the summit without your guidance and support. Humane and courageous. There are moments in the ascent of the mountain of dementia that require great courage and great humanity. Part of the Sherpa's role is to be aware of what the mountaineer needs from moment to moment. To think about them, to remember them, and at times to remember for them, to remember what they need and are likely to need. To keep them in mind. Encouragement, comfort, reality check, knowledge, validation. They cannot do this without you.

The second part of this book is an alphabetical exploration of issues that you face as a caregiver when you live with a person with dementia. Topics are cross-referenced with others related to them in *italics*.

Part I

THE RELATIONSHIP COMPASS

This brings us to the various approaches you can take when caring for a person living with dementia. As a Sherpa, you will likely take up all of these from time to time. Being in a relationship with someone, you need to be flexible. Try to avoid becoming stuck in one position or think you should be a certain type of carer or behave a certain way all the time. It may be that you have an idea of how a carer should act from watching someone you admire, or perhaps you only know of one person who has cared for a person with dementia and they did it this way, or that way, so you think you should be like that. This will only make things worse for you both and cause problems, conflicts and upsets for both of you.

If you think of a compass, there are many points around it. There are also many ways you can be with someone with dementia. On the relationship compass you will need to move around the many possible positions so that you can maintain the well-being of the person with dementia and yourself. This requires flexibility and timing to use the right position or approach at the right time. Have a look at Figure I.1.

There are many ways you can be with the person with dementia, depending on the situation. Let's look at four common scenarios. You might like to add your own combinations or relabel the positions here to make sense for your relationship.

13

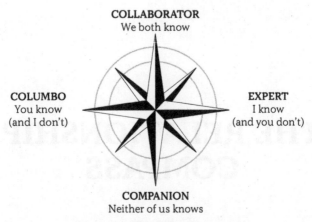

Figure I.1: *The relationship compass*

Expert – I know (and you don't)

You know what needs to be done. You know what is wrong. You understand. You can give advice. This is the 'expert' position. The person with dementia doesn't know or understand or is not seeing the risk or opportunities that you see.

There are times when the *Expert* position is necessary, such as when physical safety is at risk. The person with dementia turns to walk into traffic with no awareness of the possibility of being injured. You can see the risk and they can't. Responsibility for acting is with you to prevent them being hurt.

This is also the position when it comes to giving advice. You have knowledge and can share it. They may not have knowledge of the situation. You know that the plan for the day is to go to lunch at the golf club and this requires a rather formal standard of dress. You can suggest or tell (perhaps) the person what to wear: 'You'll need to wear a tie. That green one looks good on you.' This is the *Expert* position.

Columbo – You know (and I don't)

For those unfamiliar with the 1970's American TV character, Columbo was the bumbling cop whom villains thought of as an ignorant fool because he asked questions that showed he didn't understand. Or so they thought. He always got the crook by the end of the show. As *Columbo*, you adopt an 'I don't know' stance that values what the person with dementia thinks and wants. You apologize for not understanding. You ask questions. You seek to understand.

This is strategic. It is also the right thing to do from an ethical point of view. It values the person's preferences. Your goal here is to lift them up in the interaction by giving them importance and priority so they can contribute their perspective. They may have difficulty finding the words to explain what they want. You can ask questions that help them clarify things for themselves and for you. This is useful if you are both stuck in a disagreement about what should happen next. Often the steam will go from the interaction and you can then move to *Collaborator* with the person to find a mutually agreeable solution.

Collaborator – We both know

Collaboration can provide rare but important moments that sustain you both. You may need to hold back from being the *Expert* in order to allow the person with dementia an opportunity to use their skills and contribute knowledge so that their sense of agency and effectiveness can flourish. This is a position of collaboration in which you can work together to enjoy moments of contentment.

As dementia progresses, these moments may be less frequent and you may need to move to the *Expert* position. The person with dementia can feel relieved and calmer when you take over because it may provide them with security and a sense of safety. They are with someone who knows what to do. It is important here to do this in a manner that is gentle, calm and kind. Avoid being domineering, abrupt and bossy. That will activate either push-back or withdrawal, both of which are unpleasant and unhealthy for the person with dementia, and may damage the trust and respect in your relationship.

Companion – Neither of us knows

The *Companion* involves sitting with the person with dementia in their lack of motivation or direction or knowledge of what to do about the situation. It is the position described by Keats:

I mean Negative Capability, that is, when a man is capable of being in uncertainties, mysteries, doubts, without any irritable reaching after fact and reason. (Keats, 1899, p.277)

The *Companion* is about being present for the person with dementia. Motivation and activity are low. It can be tiring to function at such a low level of activity. It can also be anxiety-provoking to sit with the lack of direction and action. However, it can bring you together in a way that you may not normally experience when you are active and busy.

This can be a companionship that brings comfort and calmness. It is about 'being with' rather than 'doing with'.

It may be that these are the times when dementia becomes the third presence in the room. Feelings about the dementia can emerge in each of you and come to awareness. How do you each feel about this 'thing' that has changed your lives? Maybe that is what you end up doing – talking about 'not doing'.

Moving from one position to another

There will be times when you need to be flexible and think quickly to move from one approach or position to another in order to bring about success or a goal of being dressed or washed or ready to go shopping.

For example, if the person with dementia dresses in a manner inappropriate for the weather or the social situation (for example, they may be adamant that they are ready to leave for a family gathering but are dressed in underwear only), you may begin in the *Expert* position to bring it to the person's attention: 'I think you might need to put on some trousers to go to lunch.' But you cannot remain there if you get a negative response or resistance and wish to avoid upset and being late for lunch, given how certain he is that he is ready. You may need to move to the Columbo position for a moment: 'Oh, I forgot to tell you, Aunt Grace is going to be there today. She really likes those black trousers of yours/that jumper of yours. Do you think that would be good to wear? I don't know. What do you think?' Your goal is for him to be dressed appropriately. However, given the risk of upset if you impose your preferences on him, you may decide that so long as he has trousers, a shirt and a jumper on that will be okay. Which trousers doesn't really matter. To achieve this you become the *Collaborator*, who works to achieve the goal of being at the family gathering in a peaceful mood.

Why do people with dementia do the things they do?

There are many things that cause us to do the things we do. This section will examine these causes: physical health, emotions, personality, memories, trauma, psychological needs and physical environment.

People with dementia are motivated by the same needs and wants as you and me. What we say here about people with dementia is just as true for people without dementia. This is a fundamental point that is often confused by the way we speak about people with dementia. People with dementia are just people. They don't become some type of strange alien because they have a diagnosis of dementia. They are still who they were before the diagnosis. They are not mad, insane or bonkers. Some of our language has improved over the last few decades but much still needs to be done to encourage people to speak accurately and respectfully when communicating about people with dementia.

What does change in dementia is our ability to process the problems that others process automatically and therefore unconsciously (out of awareness) and work out what to do about these problems. This capacity changes gradually over time.

At its most fundamental, behaviour is anything we do or say. And what makes us behave? A stimulus, a cause. I smile at you. You smile back. I cry and you feel sad inside. Stimulus-response is a basic way of understanding behaviour. A stimulus is anything that causes you to do something, or experience something inside and then act. There is always a cause, a reason. Always. It can take some effort to identify it but it is always there.

Causes of behaviour are external and internal (see Figure I.2). External causes are those in the environment around us. The situation you are in may be causing you to feel hot, cold, calm, annoyed, sad or frustrated. You walk past a bakery at 7am, not having had your breakfast, and the smell of freshly baked bread activates your tummy to rumble. Your brain has registered the aroma, and the associations with pleasure and eating cause your stomach to release gastric juice in readiness for this tasty food. In this way, external causes can cause internal reactions. They can also cause you to interrupt your early morning walk and turn into the bakery to buy a croissant! The external cause stimulates you to act. If you think about it in terms of a sequence it may be clearer:

Smell fresh bread – stomach rumbles – enter bakery and buy croissant

External stimulus – internal experience/response – external response/behaviour

Internal causes are those we experience inside our bodies and minds. Memory, thoughts, emotions and senses all come together to create our sense of the world and what to do about it. Our brains work out what to do about it extremely quickly and efficiently.

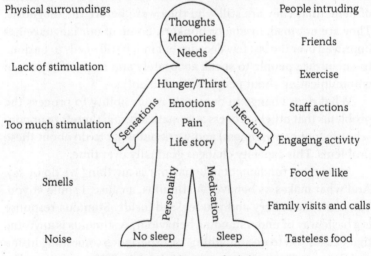

Figure I.2: Possible causes for behaviour

Physical health

Our physical health can cause us to behave in ways that can be confusing and distressing to ourselves and others. It should be the first consideration when searching for the reasons why people behave the way they do. For instance, pain can cause us to wince or become preoccupied and have difficulty concentrating on what others say to us. It can also cause us to become irritable with others. Treat the pain and the cause of the pain and the behaviour will lessen.

Strokes in particular parts of the brain can cause certain behaviour to be more likely. For instance, strokes in the right-frontal region may result in socially disinhibited behaviour and leave verbal ability intact.

Infections can cause our well-being to plummet, and require treatment with antibiotics. An example that often occurs is a urinary tract infection (UTI). This can have a rapid onset and cause changes in thinking, memory, mood and behaviour.

Hunger, thirst and other forms of physical discomfort, such as overheating or underheating, can also cause behavioural and mood changes. Identify the cause, treat it and the behaviour will lessen.

Emotions

The next consideration is emotions. If we think of it in terms of emotional moments in the day, we can see how our feelings become involved in explaining our behaviour. Our feelings have physical components and mental or psychological components. For example, when we feel upset/sad, we have a thought/image *and* a physical experience that come together to make the sadness a feeling. It may be in response to something we have seen, such as a picture of someone from our life who has died. Memories come and we feel the love we have for them still. A wave of sadness rushes up and we feel tears in our eyes, our chest and throat fill and we reach for the tissues. This is the sequence:

> We see the picture of our loved one who has died (cause/stimulus) – remember and feel the love we have for them (internal response, mental and physical) – feel a wave of sadness rising and our eyes fill with tears, our chest and throat feel full (internal response, mental and physical) – sob to release grief (behaviour response) – reach for tissues (behaviour response).

This sequence is mostly internal but is stimulated by an external object (the picture of a loved one) and also involves a box of tissues. Everything else is internal. It cannot be seen or heard by anyone else. Internal experience is private and unknowable by others until we act and reveal what is going on inside ourselves in our behaviour (crying and reaching for tissues). An onlooker may be confused by our upset, not knowing of our love for the person we have seen in the picture. They may provide comfort simply on what they can see, without knowing the internal memories and emotions that have been activated.

Personality

Extroverts seek contact with others for pleasure and enjoyment. Introverts seek time on their own for the same pleasure and enjoyment. This broad generalization holds true for many of us but usually we are a mix of both and find pleasure in contact with others and time on our own. Too much of one or the other may cause us to become irritable, tired and snappy, or to withdraw and isolate ourselves.

Some people have a personality trait of being very agreeable and others disagreeable. Some are conscientious and others couldn't care less. Some are humble and others proud, needing affirmation. Personality has an influence on how we behave.

Memories and trauma

Memories as well as emotions may cause us to behave in certain ways. As you can see from the above example, crying may be caused by memories of a loved one, which in turn activate feelings. Memories and emotion are often connected. They seem to come at once, but studies have shown that there can be a brief moment between them, and that one may cause the other. It can be either way. Memories can cause emotion. Emotions can cause memories to come. Sadness in response to a photo of a person can stimulate past losses and hurts.

This is also true for traumatic memories. Current experience can cause activation of past trauma. Memories and experience can come together to create an overwhelming moment of stress as though the past experience is happening right now. We will discuss this in some detail in Part II, *Trauma*.

Needs

Another cause for us acting or behaving in a certain way is that we experience needs. There are many models of human needs that have been developed over the last century or so. Perhaps the most well-known is Maslow's Hierarchy of Needs. We won't go into it here as there is a great deal of information on the internet about this model. Suffice to say it is a useful way to understand what motivates people to act the way they do.

When our needs are met, we tend to be calmer, more contented and less anxious, angry and acting out. When our needs are not met, we can become irritable, frustrated, angry, sad, depressed and withdrawn; we may lose confidence, or act out to get our needs met.

A model of needs was developed with people with dementia in mind by the late Tom Kitwood (1997). It consists of five basic needs: *comfort*, *occupation*, *attachment*, *identity* and *inclusion*. If we look at each need we can understand more about the motivations of people with dementia. These are universal needs that everyone experiences and they can help us understand the motivation behind much of the behaviour we see of people with dementia, and of ourselves.

Comfort

Comfort can be physical and emotional. Physical comfort may come from having enough food, a bed that is right for us, or furniture that fits us. Emotional comfort may come from affection from people we love, validation of what we are saying or from being able to trust the reliability of people who keep turning up.

Comfort may come from living in a house that is the right temperature, not too draughty or dark, or too full of glaring lights. We need a temperature that is pleasant, not too hot, not too cold, and we need to dress accordingly. However, if we are forgetful and lack awareness of our surroundings, we may go outside on a cold rainy day in a t-shirt and shorts. Or we may dress for winter weather when the day is hot and steamy, risking dehydration and sunburn.

Familiarity of our surroundings also gives comfort and soothes us. We sit in the same chair. We walk to the shops to buy the same newspaper every day for years on end. We wear that old

LIVING WITH A PERSON WITH DEMENTIA

jumper or jeans because they are comfortable, familiar. We eat food because it is familiar and satisfying. More than that, to be in familiar surroundings, clothed in familiar clothes, with familiar people is pleasurable and calming.

And this is where we confront the stresses that dementia can cause. It is difficult to be comfortable when you can't remember the people, the place, the clothing. In fact, it is more likely to be concerning and irritating. In other words, our need for comfort can be sabotaged by dementia and we can be plunged repeatedly into the discomfort of strangeness.

Personality and temperament may play a role here as we can vary in how much familiarity we need to feel comfortable. Some people thrive on new situations and enjoy wearing different clothes, engaging in novel activities and meeting new people. These people are not going to find the forgetfulness of dementia as discomforting as someone who relies on the familiarity of predictable routine for comfort.

Life experience may also influence how much comfort a person needs and what they utilize to provide that comfort. A former tradesman may want to be outside working rather than sitting inside and watching television. Then again, the former tradesman may be relieved to sit inside and be out of the weather watching his favourite football team on TV. That may be what he needs to do to signal to his brain that he can relax.

Occupation

Being occupied is important for well-being. We can take this for granted if we are employed and have structure, purpose and routine in our day. Being occupied can provide the satisfaction of making, digging, painting, folding, sorting, washing up, cooking and so much more. You get the idea. If we achieve, it is good for our self-esteem, confidence to try other things or even just to keep doing the things we do every day, which reinforces memory. This is why dressing, washing, eating and grooming are important activities to maintain for a person with dementia. As the condition progresses the person may require gradually increased assistance to achieve success but it is crucial that we do not take over. Our role is to provide the scaffolding for them to successfully perform the task themselves.

Occupation is good because it causes us to retrieve past skills from memory and use them again and again and again. This reactivates the old skills and knowledge and increases the chances of these abilities lasting longer in the face of dementia. Use it or lose it.

If we don't have the structure of someone around us prompting what is going to happen next, we can sit around waiting, feeling stuck and bored, particularly if the condition affects the motivational area of our brain. A person in this state is at risk of depression, in addition to the physical problems that can develop due to inactivity.

Boredom is a problem for some people with dementia. This usually occurs if they have difficulty initiating activity. If their 'starter motor' is not working as it used to, they may need you to prompt and prod or make suggestions. You need to work out what manner, tone and approach might get the best result. Adjust your approach until you get the right combination of words, tone and manner that prompts the person with dementia into action.

Occupation provides an opportunity to reaffirm our sense of ourselves. Who am I? I am a carpenter, a mother, a gardener, a farmer. How do I know this? Because I do the things that carpenters, mothers, gardeners and farmers do.

Attachment

Attachments are the bonds we form with people, animals, places and things. The earliest bond we form is usually with our mothers. This or a bond with another person who is our primary caregiver becomes the template for all other bonds we make in our lives. We can launch into life with a solid sense of ourselves if we make secure bonds of affection that give us an experience of safety and security.

If, however, we have early bonds that are not secure, but are unpredictable and chaotic, or harsh and punishing, this can make us anxious and worried about affection and safety, or perhaps make us want to avoid affection. We tend to form later relationships in the same way.

Making attachments is what we do as humans. So when dementia comes, we continue to form and need relationships with others, with animals, places and things. Familiar people assume a greater importance for providing a feeling of safety and calm. All the better if these people are affectionate and warm (if that is what gives us a feeling of being safe).

It is important to remember that some people may not have ever formed a sense of being safe because of early difficult childhood experiences. So they may react in their dementia from the old patterns, avoiding closeness or becoming anxious and insecure about your affection.

Attachments to animals and objects also remain important for some people. It may be a favourite chair, a worn old jumper, or a photo of their old dog or even her lead.

Thomas has been sitting quietly all afternoon in the lounge. He has slept for a good part of it, then watched daytime TV for a while. Without notice, he gets up from the chair, walks to the laundry where he grasps the dog lead off the hook and says, 'Come on then.' He goes out of the back door and into the park that backs onto his garden. Michael, Thomas's partner, discovers him gone from the lounge about 20 minutes later. He realizes what has happened, pulls on a jacket and boots, and follows him into the park. At first, he can't find him but listens and eventually he hears him calling out, 'Chloee...Chloee.' 'There you are,' Michael says.

'I can't find her, the rascal. She went haring off into the bushes after a rabbit and I lost sight of her.'

'Never mind. She'll come home when she's ready. She always does,' says Michael. Chloe is their Jack Russell terrier who died 15 years ago. Thomas had walked her in that park every day of her life and almost every day she went after rabbits, Thomas calling her and walking home with the lead in his hand. And now for the last couple of years, this is what he does when the memory takes him. Today, Michael walks alongside him and talks gently about Chloe until they are nearly home and he starts to talk about supper.

Who and what we are attached to remains important for us well beyond the moment. For some, it may be people, for others, objects or even places – former towns or homes we have lived in, people we once knew. What is significant about them is the feeling we have about those places, objects, people and animals.

It may be that an old relationship assumes a significance for a person with dementia in the present time. This can be very disturbing for you to find your spouse talking fondly about a former husband or wife. This has nothing to do with their affection for you. It has everything to do with their inability to stay in the present and the brain's need to find meaningful connection in whatever way it can. If they can't retain the present moment, old memories may be more easily accessible. So the brain follows the path of least effort and finds the old flame. Disturbing perhaps, but it doesn't mean they don't love you. They just can't hold on to you in their minds as easily as they can the long-term memories.

Identity

Who are you? How do you know who you are? Identity is a vital need we all have to know who we are. And it is jeopardized by the forgetfulness of dementia and affirmed or threatened by the way people around those with dementia treat them.

Our identity as a person is formed in the soup of relationships, memories, experiences and things that have meaning for us in our lives. Identity can be associated with our roles in life. These may be occupational roles or personal roles.

What we do or have done for work may tell us who we are. I am a carpenter because I do carpenter things. I carry and use tools. I build things. I measure, saw, hammer, screw and glue. The clothes we wear for work also tell us who we are. A carpenter may wear overalls and a beanie. An accountant may wear a suit and tie to work. A farmer may don a thick jumper and a hat in winter.

Our identity can provide us with social standing. Because of our identity role others may offer us respect in the way they speak to us, confirming a sense of ourselves. 'Hello Andy, you old bugger!' tells me that I am a friend to this person who feels fondly enough towards me to address me in a familiar way. I can now remember that my name is Andy and that I have a friend, likely an old friend. If someone addresses us as Mr, Mrs or Ms we know they do not know us well or that our relationship with them is more formal than intimate.

If someone uses a nickname or a familiar shortened version of our name it tells us about their relationship with us. They feel close to us. They know us and have some affection for us. It is worth bearing in mind that not everyone is invited into the social space where it is appropriate to use a nickname. Often it is not appropriate for a younger person to use a nickname for an older person, nor to use affectionate terms such as 'darling', 'love' or 'sweetheart'. If you are not sure, wait until you sense the nature of your relationship with them and, if possible, ask if they would be comfortable with you calling them the name. Check it out. That in itself signals respect.

Inclusion

Social inclusion is a vital need and is often thwarted by ageist exclusion or by people assuming those with dementia do not need any assistance, by forgetting, or by simply not caring. Add dementia to being older and exclusion occurs frequently. If we are included, we tend to flourish. We belong, are part of the flow of life, feel connected and alive. If we are excluded, we tend to shrivel up isolated, even in a crowded room.

When we are younger and able to converse and contribute to social engagement, inclusion is easily sustained, often to the point that we don't even notice it. We just take for granted that we are part of things. However, when we get older and have trouble sustaining conversation or have word loss or memory loss that robs us of the thread of conversation, inclusion is difficult to sustain. We can easily drop into silent watching and then disengagement. We sit silently and are somewhere else inside. Or we just settle into mental neutral. Nothing happening.

Exclusion like this is toxic for our brains. If we mentally freewheel in neutral often enough, our brains get the message that it's okay to stop working. Inactivity sends a message to our brains that there is no need for it to keep functioning so it stops. Use it or lose it.

Studies of autopsies of the brains of people diagnosed with Alzheimer's dementia have shown that even though their behaviour showed signs of memory loss and cognitive problems, a good proportion of them did not have sufficient changes in the brain to justify a diagnosis of Alzheimer's disease. They had minimized their lives to include little social engagement or physical and intellectual activity. Other study participants whose lives were rich socially and intellectually showed few signs of dementia in their lives even though their brains showed significant signs of Alzheimer's disease. What do we make of this? Some dementia appears to be due to chronic inactivity that starts in late middle age as the first signs of ageing occur, rather than due to brain pathology. Conversely, if we have lives rich with social engagement, inclusion and intellectual stimulation well into old age and do not signal to our brains that it is time to turn off, this appears to have a protective effect on brain function as we grow older. We have a good chance of maintaining our lives well into the time that any Alzheimer's disease pathology is present.

So for people with a diagnosis of dementia, it's important to maintain as much brain activity and normal functioning as possible. This means including them in everyday activities as a matter of course. If possible, try to avoid adjusting your expectations down to suit their level of activity. Stretch them with some challenges that they can succeed at with effort and scaffolding support. You are the Sherpa helping, guiding and supporting where they need it to scale the mountain.

Physical environment

Finally, the external causes of behaviour may involve the physical environment. This includes the familiarity or strangeness of the space, whether it is cluttered or spacious, the temperature, lighting, lack of opportunity for stimulation or interest, and lack of signs for way-finding. Any or all of these can cause a person with dementia to react with behaviour that signals discomfort or confusion or agitation.

A word about the brain and dementia

I am tired after working in the garden most of the day. I have had little water to drink. When my wife asks me who called earlier in the day, I can't remember the name of the friend who phoned. I have a mental block. Once I have eaten dinner, rehydrated and rested, it comes to me. It was Muhammad!

Our brains function well usually. We can remember, solve problems, plan ahead, organize ourselves to get where we want to go, see, hear, smell, taste and touch the world around us. But if we neglect our brains by having too little to drink and eat, by putting too much stress on ourselves with high workloads, or becoming ill, we can find that our brains struggle to do those everyday things for us. Or if we choose to do little into old age, making no effort to keep stimulated and engaged, we can forget, become confused, have mental blocks, make mistakes, injure ourselves, or become frustrated and explode emotionally. This can be temporary or, in the case of dementia, become worse over time. Let us now get to know the brain as it develops in a small child and what happens as we develop into adults.

Brain development

Infants soak up the world through their senses like a sponge. More than that, they experience and react to the world emotionally as they do not yet have language or thought to interact with it. There are no words, just emotions and no sense of past, present or future. It is all now. There is no time-based memory. As adults, we are so accustomed to thinking and using words that we forget that there was a time we didn't have this way of being a person.

Developing infants quickly become bonded emotionally to their main caregiver, usually the mother but not always (whoever supplies food, affection and comfort). If this bond is reliable and successful, infants grow in confidence and trust that love will come, that food will come, that comfort will come. They confirm a sense of themselves as loved. They begin life knowing emotionally that they are loved and lovable, and that the world can be trusted. Quickly they learn that if they cry food comes, comfort comes, and affection returns them to a state of calm. They are learning beings, creating patterns from experience so they can predict who to trust, what is likely to happen next, who they don't like and learn to mistrust. They learn how to be, so they can obtain food, comfort and pleasure.

Hemispheric differences

The brain consists of two halves or hemispheres that are joined in the middle, much as florets of cauliflower are part of the one head of cauliflower. Looking at it from the top, the brain has a left and a right hemisphere. The first two years of life are a time of rapid growth of neurons and connections between neurons. Then, a period of neuronal pruning takes place in which those neurons that have not been connected during this period die off. The brain consolidates and continues to grow with those neurons that remain. New connections between existing neurons proliferate, and new neurons continue to be produced throughout life, into old age.

The right hemisphere is our 'first responder'. It gives us immediate impressions in a global sense about what is happening to us or around us, not in words but in emotions and images, for example this feels bad, this feels right, this feels wrong and dangerous. It is where emotional experience takes place, where we first have a 'sense' of or emotional snapshot of things, people and experiences.

The growing infant has only this right-hemisphere facility in the first year or so of life until language and memory develop in the left hemisphere to enable it to commence thinking, remembering, talking and understanding the world, not just experiencing it.

The left hemisphere is predominantly responsible for linear, sequenced thinking, facts, figures, language production and comprehension and, of course, conscious memory. This is the 'logistics centre' that enables the growing infant to make sense of the flood of impressions and emotional storms that engulf it as it grapples with 'No' and 'Don't do that' from caregivers who sense risks the child cannot yet perceive or manage.

As it learns to stand up and move about, new opportunities and risks enter the life of this dynamo of a child. It is now limited by the people who previously only provided love and food and comfort and are now concerned about safety. Emotionally the infant is now faced with managing conflicting emotions, making sense of negative responses and feelings, and learning that it is loved through it all. Hopefully. The left hemisphere helps it to manage this increasing complexity, have thoughts to make sense of and understand the emotional storms that assail it and find the words to express this experience.

Emotions

We feel emotions physically. The most common way we experience emotional upset is in our bodies. Anger can be experienced as heat, muscles becoming stronger and an urge to bang or strike out. Sadness can rise in waves in our chest, fill us and then billow out in tears, with sobbing and a runny nose. Sadness can be physically painful, especially in the chest and throat. Guilt can be felt as a tightening in the throat and upper chest. Love can be felt in the chest as a rising wave, in the eyes, and in an urge to move towards another person.

Accompanying these physical sensations are the thoughts that help us interpret the physical experience. There is micro-second (about half a second) difference in time with thoughts following the physical sensation. We tend to speak of thinking in relation to feeling rather than feelings. This is most obvious when television reporters ask questions of distraught witnesses:

Reporter: How did you feel?
Witness: I thought I was going to die.

The reporter is not interested in how the person feels. They just want the sound-bite for the evening news. And the witness goes straight to thoughts rather than feelings, as if that thought is what they felt.

If we do not like feeling emotion and have developed patterns of emotional avoidance or anxiety about emotions, we may develop a tendency for emotions to cause physical pain or discomfort. In other words, we become anxious about feelings. For those with anxiety as their primary pattern, it may be in muscle tightness (chest pain, joint pain or muscle aches, spasms and cramps) and headaches or migraines.

For those whose main pattern is to avoid emotional closeness, this can physically manifest in migraine, asthma-type shortness of breath, gastrointestinal problems and headaches. It is important to have these medically examined to exclude physical illness as the cause, rather than assume it is emotionally driven.

Emotions and the brain

Emotions are like the skin with which we sense the world. Initially, the growing infant has only emotions to respond to what it senses and experiences. Being fed, loved and made comfortable is all it needs. It learns who it feels good with, who meets its needs, who limits it, who misses the mark, who it has to be quiet with, who makes it feel worse/better. It learns how it has to be to be accepted and loved. It makes emotional sense of this new world it experiences. So it comes to develop an emotional identity. *This is how they are with me so this must be who I am and this is how the world is. I am accepted when I am quiet. I get love when I am good. I am okay when I don't have anger. When I don't show anxiety, she is happy. When I don't cry, she stays happy.*

Initially, the infant cannot regulate its own emotions and relies on its caregiver to manage its emotions by responding to its distress in good time, by giving it the right amount of milk/nourishment, by sensing when it has had enough, by providing a clean nappy, by limiting or correcting and loving at the same time. Over time, the growing infant learns to regulate its emotions itself. It develops a sense of a good emotional state that feels right (homeostasis) and learns how that state is associated with its caregiver and others. This becomes its identity or sense of self and it is developed in relationship with important others such as parents or other caregivers. Most of the time it is sufficient to enable the growing child to develop into a functioning human, able to become a healthy effective parent and contributor to society. Or not.

Not all parenting is skilled and successful, or reliable. Sometimes it is damaging. Unfortunately, many children grow through infancy and into childhood with little affection, and untimely and punitive reactions from parents. Or they endure years of emotional inconsistency from parents or other caregivers whose own needs dominate. Children get the message that they are nuisances, that they don't matter, that they have to be invisible, or that they have to be pretty, or clever, or silent and invisible, or nice to get love. The effect usually endures into adulthood unless the growing person has the good fortune to be loved by a partner who can heal the wounds of childhood, or meet a therapist who can help them.

Many grow into adults who avoid intimacy because emotional

closeness activates emotions and associated memories that are too painful. Closeness is avoided. Many spend a lifetime avoiding closeness to others by being intellectually focused, brusque and angry, or detached, depressed and disinterested. Many become anxious, worried about closeness and preoccupied about whether they are loved. They question who loves them and what they have to do to be loved. Yet they do not feel really seen for who they are because they are deeply afraid they will not be loved. So, they swing between wanting to be close and wanting to be invisible.

Most of us have some memories of childhood or specific emotional experiences that are painful, in addition to the pleasant ones. We don't want to dig them up. The changes brought about by dementia often activate these old memories and emotions, which can be confusing and disorienting for people with dementia. The past can become confused with the present, as the feelings are activated as if the past is happening now.

Emotions have no clock, no past, present or future. All the brain knows is what it is experiencing right now. Regardless of whether an event happened in the past, the emotional experience is as if it is now. The right hemisphere, where early emotional experience occurs in images and physical states, has no time attached to it. It is all present moment until language comes along at about 12–24 months of age when children gradually develop a sense of now, later, not yet, yesterday and tomorrow.

So, for a person with dementia, the fact that a feeling is activated now, but originates from a past experience, may be lost on them. It is just now. As a caregiver, you must try to maintain a sense of mental distance at times that can enable you to be a calming presence rather than becoming caught up in it or seeming defensive and making it worse. This mental distance ideally can accompany the capacity to be present in the moment for the person you are with. There just needs to be a corner of your mind that is watching yourself interacting.

However, you too will have your own personal history of childhood and growing up with perhaps less than ideal parenting, and your own legacy of emotional avoidance or anxiety about closeness. So...be patient with yourself. This is discussed in more detail in the section 'Attachment, caregiving and dementia'.

Foundations – what behaviour is

Behaviour is anything we do or say. It is visible or audible. It is what others can see or hear from us.

Behaviour is not what goes on inside a person. That is thought or emotion and is not visible or audible. It may be linked to it but it is different. Studies have shown that there is a half-second delay between a thought and action, between a feeling and action, so the brain can register a feeling or a thought and then it causes a physical reaction.

Behaviour is a form of communication to others about what is going on inside us. Crying is behaviour that usually communicates sadness or distress. Aggression usually communicates anger or a response to fear. Hugging may communicate affection or love.

It can also tell others about ourselves. Our behaviour shows others what we like, prefer or want, or dislike and don't want. It can tell others how something has affected us. Crying shows we are sad about something, perhaps what someone has done to us, or we are sad that we can't do something we like doing.

Behaviour is meaningful. So when you look at what a person you care for is doing, you need to ask yourself what they intend or mean by the behaviour. This question is the basic building block of understanding the other person. Ask 'why?' What is the reason they changed in mood from calm to agitated as the afternoon progressed? What does this mean?

ABC model of behaviour

The ABC model is a simple approach to understanding behaviour in which A = *Antecedent*, B = *Behaviour* and C = *Consequence*. It is widely used to focus attention on the causes and consequences of behaviour in order to understand what is causing and maintaining the behaviour.

It is often oversimplified to focus on only one cause or antecedent and one consequence. This ignores the complexity of human behaviour. Usually, multiple factors must be considered to truly understand why a person acts a certain way in a particular situation. If this model is to be used, it must be in the broadest terms so that the many possible causes and consequences are included.

It is important also to work out whether it is the antecedents (A) or consequences (C) that are maintaining the behaviour (B). In this way, you can target your energy to the factors that are going to have the most effect. For instance, if a person with dementia is consistently refusing to cooperate with eating their evening meal, it may be that lunch is too large and their previous meal is still giving them a sense of fullness (antecedent), or it may be that they have learned that if they refuse long enough you will give them dessert first (consequence). If it is the size of lunch, you can alter portion size. If it is dessert that encourages refusal of the main course, your efforts may need to go to not offering dessert but instead letting the person experience hunger until they engage with the evening meal in their own time.

Offering a reward (C) works if the person can sustain a memory of being promised the reward long enough to do the behaviour (B). If there is a time lapse (such as minutes, hours or days depending on the individual), the person may forget the reward that was promised. So, for someone with forgetfulness, using consequences may not be helpful or effective.

Behaviour change

You can change behaviour in several ways. Using consequences as noted above is one way. Other ways include reasoning, negative consequences to decrease the frequency of a behaviour, limit setting and distraction. Negative consequences to decrease a behaviour are forms of punishment. I strongly urge you not to use punishment when in a caring relationship with a person with dementia. I mention it only for completeness as it has been used in many 'behaviour modification' programmes historically. It is not consistent with a respectful person-centred approach to relating with another person in a caregiving relationship. People with dementia often have little enough in their lives without us taking more from them or introducing something noxious to make them move away from it.

Reasoning may or may not be useful. It depends on the person's capacity to participate in the reasoning conversation, their memory capacity, the situation and the importance of the behaviour to them and to you. I suggest that using reasoning requires more problem-solving and abstract thinking ability than many people with dementia have a capacity for. I encourage you to not engage in using this method of changing behaviour.

That said, it depends on the person with dementia. If they are able to reason and you can do it without dominating the person, then use it. But be wary of using reasoning as your 'go to' approach. I often hear carers say, 'I tried to reason with him but...' Usually, you find that emotional needs overwhelm logic and you will be back where you started, now with a person in a defensive mood.

Limit setting is useful, particularly if you keep it simple, if the limit makes some sense to the person with dementia and if the limit is reasonable and in proportion to the behaviour of concern. For example, you might say, 'We can have two biscuits each.'

Distraction is low on the totem pole of desirable behaviour change approaches. It is frequently used as a quick and effective way that requires little from you and often gives instant success in changing a person's behaviour. The reason it is less desirable is that it can be used instead of approaches that take time and more thought and effort.

Attachment, caregiving and dementia

Behavioural disturbance in dementia can be referred to as distress behaviour (see Part II, *Distress behaviour*). It is reasonable to refer to much of it as attachment distress behaviour. It is generally activated by insecurity or anxiety. Why does this happen when the person has lived a full, confident adult life and not shown insecurity or dependence on others?

Attachment is a bond that people and animals form with caregivers who provide food, affection and security. It is most often seen in infant behaviour towards parents but continues throughout life into old age. It is seen in seeking, calling out, distress at separation, relief when the caregiver is nearby. You see it in displays of affection and closeness between life-long partners.

Dementia activates attachment behaviour. Bere Miesen and Gemma Jones identified attachment behaviour in people with dementia in their book *Caregiving in Dementia* (1992): wanting to go home, to go to parents, to have a parent's attention, to worry about parents, to imagine themselves back in the childhood home

LIVING WITH A PERSON WITH DEMENTIA

with parents, acting like a good girl/boy, feeling threatened by parental authority, and asking where parents are.

The person with dementia can experience a 'strange situation' as they move through their day, forgetting things and being unable to hold people in mind. Moments disappear out of memory. The 'strange situation' term was coined to describe the research experience that Mary Ainsworth set up for infants and mothers. The mother entered a room with the baby. Then the mother left and the baby was on its own and then a stranger entered, left after a time, and finally the mother returned. All the while, the reactions of the baby were noted. This is where the patterns of secure, anxious and avoidant behaviour were first identified.

The strange situation of dementia activates the attachment behaviour of seeking security and safety, through contact or by avoidance. Withdrawal can look like the absence of distress. However, avoidance of closeness by withdrawing is essentially a distress management strategy. The person with dementia may also withdraw by shutting down emotionally as a reaction to a need for the parent. In an infant, this shutdown is the infant's attempt to protect itself from being emotionally hurt by inappropriate parental behaviour such as absence, overly intense compensation following absence, parental dominance or punishment. Inconsistent parenting is as problematic for childhood attachment, as is absent or neglectful parenting. Dementia activates these old patterns.

Essentially, when dementia occurs the person can feel insecure, anxious and uncertain at times due to difficulty responding to day-to-day problems that require thinking or remembering. Anxiety about making mistakes and/or grief and frustration about not being able to do things that were previously easy to do are activated in these moments. This emotional distress then causes the person to seek comfort and reassurance, or to move away and avoid others, depending on what their usual pattern of managing feelings has been. This can be confusing and angering for a caregiver, as it may be different from how you have known them. But if we understand it through the lens of attachment, we can build a clear picture of what is going on and take some of the confusion and upset out of it.

When attachment distress is experienced we generally act in one of three typical patterns, or a mix of these patterns: security, anxiety or avoidance. Over the past 90 years, this has been studied widely and there is a huge body of evidence to support this way of looking at attachment behaviour.

Secure attachment

Security is the pattern that happens when a person is capable of being reassured and returns to calm when they feel challenged or disturbed by emotional upset or difficulties. They tend to seek help when they need it. The secure person can utilize help to return to a calm, contented state. They can be guided without feeling stressed about it. This person can handle new situations without feeling overwhelmed with anxiety or backing off and withdrawing from challenges. Essentially, they are secure in themselves and face life with confidence and contentment.

Anxious attachment

The second pattern of attachment behaviour is an anxious/preoccupied pattern seen in a tendency to worry about whether they are loved and remembered by others. They can have difficulty trusting reassurance once this worry comes to mind. The anxiously attached person can tend to seek out reassurance but not find it effective. It is easy to recognize the list that Miesen and Jones put together in this style of coping with the strange situation of dementia. The anxiously attached person can also worry or be preoccupied about their abilities, overwhelmed and ashamed by their mistakes and unable to shift out of this painful mood. They tend to seek out closeness or proximity to others for security, particularly others who are emotionally important, but when the chips are down anyone will do!

However, contentment is elusive, as the old anxiety is usually not healed. In life, a person may heal the old wounds of childhood if they have a life partner who helps them to heal or if they are fortunate to engage in psychotherapy that goes a little deeper than the usual approaches. But dementia can reactivate old emotional insecurities and overwhelm whatever healing was achieved earlier in life.

Avoidant attachment

The third pattern is avoidance. In this pattern, people tend to move away from others when they feel emotionally upset. They have their pain on their own. In its most extreme form, they can avoid closeness at all times and live behind a shield of defensiveness, seen in patterns of formality or rigidity that make being close to this person difficult. They seldom feel love or affection and this is the purpose of their defensiveness. To not feel anything is the goal. They can be dismissive of attempts to be close or affectionate. If you can't feel love or affection then you can't feel hurt or pain when love doesn't come or can't be relied on, or when caregiving is harsh and punishing, as it is for children sometimes.

It is important to make clear that these patterns of behaviour are common in human and animal behaviour. We all display some of these traits from time to time. When dementia affects people's lives, these patterns become more obvious and affect their day-to-day life more dramatically.

Increases in dependency due to difficulty remembering (for instance, what we said we would do today) and working out how to handle situations (something as mundane as getting dressed) can cause explosions of rage and shame, which can then be followed by regretful sadness and bursts of crying or avoidant moody withdrawal. People who are anxious in their main pattern of attaching to others can be explosive or overwhelmed and in tears easily. People who are avoidant as their main pattern are more likely to simply move away, or go silent and withdraw into themselves. Or they may explode if they feel emotion they can't manage, and then move away emotionally.

Dementia can reactivate old psychological wounds. The avoidance that was used in the past may re-emerge as a familiar way to deal with painful early wounds that can be felt again in the strangeness of life with dementia.

Attachment and caregiving

You are an attachment figure. In adult relationships attachments are often mutual. This occurs normally when in a life-long relationship we transfer to our partners the emotional dependency and affection we once felt towards our primary caregivers. This may be why it is sometimes said we are attracted to people who are like our father or mother! Usually the same patterns of attachment are evident throughout our lives. Each partner becomes both the attached and the caregiver. But when one partner has dementia that can change, as their ability to be a caregiver diminishes and they assume a dependent role in the relationship. This shift can be gradual and cause significant grief and resentment as the former relationship of mutual loving and caring is lost and replaced by one-way caregiving.

Patterns of attachment-distress in dementia may be seen in the characteristic support seeking or avoidance noted above. In caregiving, the person with dementia can transfer onto you the same need for security and safety they felt in relationship with their parents as a young child. This involves the same emotional template they developed in response to this early experience. In other words, you may be treated as though you are the parent figure.

This template holds expectations of the parent. It is what they came to expect as normal in their infancy. If the parent was inconsistent and intrusive, anxious about whether they were loved themselves and flipped from being overly affectionate in ways that smothered the child, to moody and withdrawn, this may have set up in the child an expectation that the way to belong in this family is to be clingy, needy and insecure. Alternatively, if the parent was emotionally absent and dismissive of the child's emotional needs, the child may have grown to avoid or shut down emotions as the way to be present in this family.

In dementia, these patterns can be activated in relation to you as the caregiver – anxiously needy or emotionally avoidant and withdrawn.

In an anxious pattern of distress management this may take the form of following, shadowing or clinging to you as their insecurity overwhelms their confidence in themselves. They can ask questions repeatedly, not really listening to the answer but filled with the question and the anxiety that the question gives them: 'Where am I?', 'When do I go home?', 'Where is Mum?' The insecurity can seem limitless and your reassurance ineffective.

In an avoidant pattern of attachment, the person with dementia may treat you as a punishing parent figure who they are angry with, they may deny they have a need for your support or assistance and push you away, resentful of your attempts at closeness and repeated attempts to ensure their safety. They may take risks because of this denial, needing rushed interventions to rescue them, which in turn can cause explosions of rage and shame.

Responses and strategies to avoid

Reasoning

I sometimes hear caregivers say, 'I tried explaining to him why he couldn't go out at this hour', or, 'I tried reasoning with her but she wouldn't listen.' These are moments of intense frustration for the caregiver and the person being cared for.

Reasoning is commonly and mistakenly used when people with dementia express an intention to do something that is based on a delusion (see *Delusions*). A delusion is a fixed false idea or thought. The person is usually not open to persuasion.

Reasoning might be useful with an adult who is able to engage with you, follow the thread of your logic and hold the abstract concepts in memory long enough for the penny to drop. Plato and Aristotle loved these approaches to argument and persuasion. If a = b and b = c, then a = c. Logical. But also abstract. It involves being clear in your mind why you are doing something and then letting go of this and changing your mind. It requires capacity for abstraction, sufficient memory capacity, mental flexibility and capacity to concentrate. It is therefore not likely to be an effective way to ensure the physical or emotional safety of a person with dementia.

Why is it not likely to be effective? Because by engaging in a reasoning exercise you are asking the person with dementia to use their thinking ability, which is compromised. They may want something that you do not want to happen, and contend with you in your efforts to change their mind. Changing one's mind is not easy at the best of times. Dementia can make it difficult for people to change their minds. If they have this difficulty, then asking them to reason is only going to raise the frustration level and increase the likelihood of an angry outburst or moody withdrawal.

Emotion is also the most common motivator that is ignored by reasoning. Maybe the person with dementia just wants to do

THE RELATIONSHIP COMPASS

something but can't be clear about it verbally, or cannot handle the effort of listening and comprehending your words when all they want is to meet a felt need.

An example of this may be seen in a story about Sarah, who some of you may remember from my first book.

Sarah has a strong sense of her own purpose and enjoys being with others in the nursing home. She comes to lunch one day after attending the hairdresser with her underwear over her tracksuit. She is carrying her handbag, and has her hair freshly coiffed. She clearly feels good about how she looks as she walks into the dining room for lunch. One of the carers approaches her and quietly says, 'Sarah, you have your undies over the top of your tracksuit.' But this attempt at reasoning is lost on Sarah, who is convinced that she is correctly dressed. She replies, 'That's how we wear them here.'

Reasoning does not work here because Sarah is firmly convinced that she is right. To force the issue would send her into a negative emotional state and potentially one in which she feels angry, ashamed or embarrassed for having made a mistake. If you force the issue, there is only one winner and that is you. The person with dementia loses. Avoid this.

Another example of a moment in which reasoning is often used is when a person with dementia wants to go home and they are already home with you.

Joan and Charles have been married for 53 years when Joan develops memory problems and becomes confused about where she is. Increasingly as the afternoons wear on she forgets who Charles is and that they have been married for most of their lives. One afternoon, Joan has been quiet for some time and Charles goes to find her in the house. He eventually finds her packing a suitcase on their bed, preparing to 'go home'. Charles has seen this before and he sits on the bed and gently says, 'But darling, you live here with me. We've been married for over 50 years and we have three lovely children together.' Joan looks up at him and says 'Don't be ridiculous' and keeps packing.

LIVING WITH A PERSON WITH DEMENTIA

Reasoning here about the facts of their lives together makes no difference to Joan. So Charles is faced with a choice. He can push on with the facts, peppering her with their children's names and stories about them and things they have done together over the years. It may stimulate a return to the present for Joan. Or it may not. If it doesn't work, he risks her becoming upset with his attempts to persuade her out of leaving the house. If this is his usual style of interacting with Joan it may initiate a cascade of resentment that has lain simmering for decades, out of which she may respond, 'Stop badgering me!' In this case, any attempt at rapport will be unsuccessful until she is calm.

If a person with dementia has a false or delusional belief, do not try to persuade them out of it with logic. It is usually fruitless and may result in rupture to the relationship. So avoid reasoning in the face of delusional beliefs.

The appropriate response for Charles is to validate Joan, and this will be examined in detail under its own heading (*Validation*) in Part II. You may wish to look ahead to that now. Or you can wait till we get there.

If her delusional belief involves her walking into danger, such as crossing a busy road, clearly Charles should intervene to ensure her safety. However, if it does not involve immediate threat of physical danger, validate and monitor for changes to physical safety.

Advice giving

I don't know about you but there are few people in my life I feel sufficiently comfortable with for them to give me advice. It depends on the circumstances, of course.

If you are reading this book, it is likely that the issues you deal with in caregiving include the mental inflexibility of a person with dementia. Dementia can cause increased difficulty in taking on other perspectives. What makes us more inflexible is attempts to persuade us or give advice that is not asked for and is therefore unwanted.

So, I suggest that gently asking questions about the situation with the person is going to be more acceptable to them than overt attempts to persuade them out of their point of view or intended action.

For instance, if they want to go home to their mother, believing that she is waiting for them at home, avoid confronting them with realities such as the fact that their mother is deceased and has been for 20 years. Such an act is likely to aggravate any need for their mother, which may increase the need to be with them. Grief and anger may surge to the surface, followed by resentment at your attempts to restrict them from going home.

However, if you were to quietly ask questions about who is at home, when they were home last, what they will do when they get home, how it feels to be home, what they used to do at home, you may have more chance of gaining more information about the motive for going home and of understanding it better. You may also offer comments about how good it feels to be at home (if that's the feeling that is suggested by the person with dementia), and draw them to talk about their mother and their life together at home. Being understood is likely to calm the person. Being restricted is not.

Consequences

We are confronted by consequences every day in our lives. The use of consequences to modify behaviour is an old method that, along with limit setting, is frequently used by parents with teenagers and young children. We do something that offends someone and we feel guilty. That's a consequence. Whether we intended it or not it is important to experience guilt when we have harmed another person. It is often a stimulus for us to remedy the wrong and make restitution or repair the relationship with an apology.

For consequences to be an effective method of behaviour change they need to be repeated, consistent and memorable. The first two criteria are possible as they depend on the behaviour of the caregiver. However, memory is impaired for people with dementia and this is what makes it difficult and perhaps ill-advised to use consequences in dementia caregiving. The person's capacity to remember is likely to be limited, depending on the individual and your relationship with them. It is much preferred to use the wide range of options to modify behaviour that you have available rather than use consequences when relating with people with dementia.

The other element to take into consideration is that the use of consequences usually involves unpleasant consequences as a discouragement for target behaviour. People with dementia are at risk of experiencing enough negative emotion without introducing negative experience as a deliberate strategy. Rather, draw the person towards the desired goal or behaviour with a specific reward. This is preferable to using a negative to draw them away from the undesired behaviour. Carrot rather than stick. Honey rather than vinegar.

You can utilize the capacity of the person with dementia to learn, in order to draw the person towards the behaviour you want more of. Reward the healthy choice and do not reward the unhealthy choice. Sometimes this means ignoring the undesirable behaviour (if you can, if it is not to do with safety) and rewarding the desired behaviour as soon as and every time it occurs until it is established. This desired behaviour replaces the undesired behaviour because they can't both occur at the same time. To make this work you must identify the reward that you are going to use. It must be specific and meaningful to the person with dementia.

The following scenario is an example of rewarding a healthy choice.

Ned is usually well groomed and his personal hygiene is excellent. However, as his dementia progresses he begins to resent taking a shower each day and reacts angrily to his wife Rose when she suggests it. Recently, he has been a week without a shower and he has begun to smell bad. Rose tells him he smells bad and he becomes angry and storms off into the workshop.

Several days later, Rose decides to try another approach. She arranges for her and Ned to have coffee with their friends Eric and Emily at the local cafe. Ned likes these people and Rose knows he enjoys Emily's company. When she let Ned know so he could get ready she says, 'You might be sitting next to Emily today.' She uses this as a 'pull' to draw Ned to take a shower, which he does. She doesn't need to supervise the showering and dressing, so when he emerges from the bathroom she compliments him on how handsome and tall he is, how good he looks, and on his aftershave. He beams as she pats the lapels of his jacket.

Rose uses the reward of the prospect of sitting next to Emily, and praise to stroke his self-esteem so he will be more likely to take a shower next time she asks him to. Using comments like this, with warmth and affirmation, Rose is more likely to have success in maintaining Ned's hygiene and consequently his ability to socialize comfortably. She links showering with the good feeling he experiences when she praises him for being handsome and tall and smelling nice. Whatever the behaviour and whatever the reward, this principle of rewarding the desired behaviour is a fundamental building block of a good behavioural approach in dementia care. It continues to work well into the moderate periods of dementia change. It is also positive as opposed to the traditional use of negative consequences and so is much more desirable.

Behavioural approaches to use

Substitution

If a person is engaging in an undesirable behaviour using an object, you can substitute something else and engage them in a more desirable and less risky behaviour.

> Jacob has been sitting in the lounge chair for two hours and he is bored. Jacob's wife Rachel has been busy with housework and has left Jacob watching television in the lounge room. He has moderate dementia and is enjoying the afternoon programmes. After an hour or so, he begins to bang his hands on the arms of the chair, making a loud noise. He keeps it up for several minutes until his wife comes in and gently puts a cushion in his lap and his hands on the cushion. He begins to bang his hands on the cushion with almost no sound.

Substituting the cushion for the arms of the lounge chair resolved the noisy disruption of Jacob's loud behaviour. The next step is to stop the housework long enough to engage Jacob in something else or have him cooperate with Rachel by doing some of the housework himself.

Another example is if a person with dementia picks up a knife and you know they do not have the awareness to use it safely.

Offer them a cup to hold instead: 'Jacob, could you help me with this cup?'

Distraction/Redirection

An approach that is commonly used as a first-line response to behavioural disruptions is distraction or redirection of attention. It's a 'Hey, look over there' strategy. I regard this as a low-grade strategy that is effective in the short term. It is low-grade because it doesn't address the causes of the behaviour. Rather, it's a sticking-plaster on the problem.

That said, it is usually effective because it interrupts the person's attention or flow and so stops the behaviour in the short term and offers the caregiver some temporary relief of stress. This usually doesn't last very long before the behaviour starts again because the cause has not been addressed.

> Mavis is repeatedly asking her husband where she is. She has been asking since breakfast and it is now mid-afternoon. She is becoming increasingly distressed with each repetition. His response is usually, 'You're home, darling. You live with me. I'm your husband Derek.' It is if she hasn't heard him. Finally, Derek remembers the draughts board. For some reason that he doesn't understand, Mavis gets great pleasure from draughts and is able to play it for several hours. He sets it up and she comes to the dining table and makes the first move.

Distraction is also useful in response to repetitiveness. Repetitiveness (see Part II) is one of the most stressing behaviours for caregivers that people with dementia can engage in. It usually occurs because the person with dementia is discontented and disturbed. Distraction is a useful short-term strategy because it disrupts attention, but you must address the causes if you wish to minimize the distress for the person with dementia and for you.

Derek successfully distracts Mavis from her preoccupation with knowing where she is. It is temporary, but it relieves his growing sense of despair that he is running out of patience and ideas.

If someone is preoccupied with 'home' and wants to know where they are, it is important to think it through to find possible causes. This specific issue will be explored in the topic in Part II, *Home*.

The guidelines for working out possible causes for behaviour are explained in 'Why do people with dementia do the things they do?' earlier in this book.

Here is another example of distraction:

> David is pulling out all the linen from the linen cupboard in an effort to find his battery drill. He is firmly convinced that his wife Maureen has hidden it from him and is annoyed and determined to find it. Maureen has stayed out of his way because she knows he is annoyed with her. In desperation, she puts on a YouTube video of a woodworker building a cupboard. She knows this always calms him as he concentrates on it for an hour or so. He hears it and walks into the lounge, sits and is focused on the program, having disconnected from his preoccupation with the lost drill. This gives her time to repack the linen cupboard and try to find his drill, which he has likely misplaced in the workshop.

The difficult behaviour is replaced by drawing the person with dementia towards a more desirable behaviour.

A popular distraction is food. It works for most of us. It is short term but it gives relief and time for everyone to reset. Finger-food is a most effective form of distraction as the person is not given a large meal but is offered small amounts of food at a time that can be managed without utensils. If they are not getting much exercise, large amounts of food can be a problem for excess weight gain. It can also be a problem if the person has diabetes or other medical conditions that limit the type or amount of food that is healthy for them (see *Finger-food*).

You may distract the person with dementia in helping you with domestic tasks. This is a non-gender activity that can help them to be occupied and productive. Depending on the skills and self-awareness of the person, they may be able to complete the tasks without too much supervision. However, you will need to use your knowledge of what they can and cannot do to scaffold (see *Scaffolding*) them so they can be successful. Scaffolding is simply providing enough of the right support to enable the person with dementia to be successful. Not too much and not too little.

Sometimes all you have to do to interrupt the person's behaviour is to touch them gently or make eye contact to gain their attention and then follow up with a lead-in to an activity or food.

What is commonly known as wandering (it is really just walking, but when people with dementia do it, it is called wandering) (see *Wandering*) is sometimes a target for distraction techniques. Distraction can be useful here if you need to interrupt the walking for health or safety reasons, for example if the person is at risk of becoming dehydrated or walking away from you and becoming lost. As above, food, activity or a gentle touch can be enough to interrupt a person's preoccupation or repetitiveness.

Distraction is always a short-term measure, but that may be what you need in the moment. It must always be used alongside more thorough planning and thinking about the causes of behaviour. Otherwise, you will be constantly going from spot fire to spot fire using distraction like a fire extinguisher when what you need is a fire-prevention strategy.

Limit setting

Limits are a natural part of life and they can be a useful tool for modifying behaviour for teenagers and young children as they learn to interact with the world. However, limits are of little value unless you already have rapport with the person. Limit setting relies on a level of trust and acceptance from the person with dementia. For a limit to be accepted, they must trust you. Limits must be delivered in a warm/neutral tone so that the limits are not misinterpreted as punishment.

An example of this is food. Perhaps the person with dementia eats to excess and you can see this is unhealthy for them. A simple way to say it is 'Tom, you can have one more sandwich' or 'Tom, why don't you have one more sandwich?' The question is less likely to aggravate but also less likely to be successful than the statement delivered as a fact.

However, an even better solution is to not put out as many sandwiches and so limit consumption by limiting the number of sandwiches the person with dementia can see. If you don't want them to eat as much, make less food available. If they keep going to the fridge, don't store as much food in the fridge. Avoid putting a lock on the fridge (I have seen this done) as it is an added cause of frustration and may cause them to say they are being kept in a prison.

Another example is, 'You can't pee in the kitchen.' It's a statement of fact. Keep it simple. Don't argue. Then give the desired behaviour. 'You can pee in the toilet/bathroom. It's here', and show the person where it is. If they are peeing in the kitchen because they are forgetting where the toilet/bathroom is, you can make signs that you can teach them to associate with locating the toilet (see *Way-finding*). Teaching them to associate the sign with peeing and toilet may take a week or so but it is possible. The success of this will depend on the capacity of the person with dementia to learn and your capacity to teach it. If you doubt your ability to teach it you may ask your local dementia support group to help you.

Stimulus control

This is a fancy name for managing how much noise or other stimulation the person is exposed to (see *Stimulation*). It is not just about limiting the stimulation but also providing selected stimulation that provides pleasure and enjoyment associated with specific memories.

It is common for people with dementia to become overwhelmed from time to time, sometimes regularly, and usually later in the day. All these situations are a call for you to manage the amount of stimulation they experience. You and I can realize we are becoming overwhelmed and do something about it. We can leave the room, leave the shopping centre, have a meal, turn the temperature down on the heating, or turn the volume down on the television.

Stimulus control is essential when you are caring for someone with dementia, and it is more often your responsibility to notice it and do something about it, as the person with dementia may not be able to recognize that they are overwhelmed or heading in that direction.

Think of each of the senses and this will give you an idea of what to look for. Each sense can be overwhelmed by stimulation:

touch, taste, smell, hearing and vision. We can also add the vestibular sense (awareness of movement). Too much touch may be overwhelming for someone who is not comfortable with a lot of touch or even a little touch. A massage is not going to be their favourite way to relax. On the contrary, they may become agitated and disturbed by such an activity.

Too much sweet, sour, salty, bitter or umami taste may be agitating. If the person is older, their taste buds may require more of specific tastes to be pleasurable (for example, if they are accustomed to salty food, they may need more salt to feel it is a tasty meal).

Normal cooking smells may have a pleasant effect and draw the person to the table ready to eat. Too much of any strong smell can cause an agitated reaction that you may think is out of proportion. Examples of this may include perfume, bleach, faeces, vomit or urine.

Loud noises can agitate older people, as can high pitched noises such as the voices of small children. Family visits of grandchildren may be welcome and give a lot of pleasure but may also agitate if allowed to go on for too long. Shorter visits may be more appropriate, with children asked to remember that grandpa or grandma really needs them to use their 'inside voice'.

The visual stimulation of shopping malls can be overwhelming for people with dementia. Bright lights, bright colours, flashing lights, lots of movement of people. Combine that with the sounds of many people talking at once, music that changes from shop to shop, crying babies and children and it produces a cacophony that is too much for the brain to process. You don't need to have dementia to find this too much to bear! Brief exposure to the visual and auditory stimulation of a shopping mall will likely be better than an extended shopping day. Plan ahead and have in mind what you are going to visit, when you will have a break and where you will sit for that break, where the toilets are and how far it is to your car.

Routine

Routine and structure are valuable in supporting the person with dementia to experience their days positively and peacefully. The benefit of routine is that the brain doesn't have to expend as much energy and effort on processing routine activities as it does on new or changing activities.

Structure is just that. You need enough regularity to permit the person to feel that they know what is coming next. This is crucial for us all. The familiarity of a regular routine enables the person to relax and enjoy the specific content of the day. The structure is like the skeleton and the activity is the meat on the bones.

Have in mind periods of activity and periods of quiet or rest, with regular breaks for food and drink. You will notice that your day is usually punctuated with these elements anyway, but with a person with dementia you may need to be more conscious of it as they may not be as able to support themselves in creating or sustaining structure in their day as you are.

An example of structure to a day may begin with toilet/bathing/showering and dressing, followed by breakfast, then a walk if the weather is fine. Then wash dishes and clean the kitchen. Then an hour outside in the garden, a break for drink and food, an indoor activity/game, lunch at home or in a cafe, an afternoon rest in the lounge or on the bed for an hour, then a drink and food, another game/reading/TV, drink and food, watch the evening news together, prepare for bed. Sounds pleasant? Yes, it does. However, it may work one day and not the next, so try to be flexible and have options that can fill a change in plans. One routine may be filled with a specific game or TV programme or other activity or friends you visit. On another day it may be a planned activity group at the local Alzheimer's centre.

The rhythm of regular activity followed by rest is important in maintaining energy levels. So are regular food and drink. Watch for flagging concentration or focus and increasing agitation. If you know the person with dementia well, you will know their signs of a dip in energy. If they need a rest sooner than the planned end of the activity, be prepared to stop what you are doing and go with the changed need. That is always the priority. You will notice that parents who have trouble with their children in supermarkets are usually those trying to impose what they want on the toddler rather than going with the child's needs for attention, energy support or a quiet break in the car to settle. Often, of course, parents have no choice but to have the cantankerous child with them as they have no back-up, and no option but to do the shopping right now as that is the only time it can be done. So too, you may find yourself in situations that spiral downward very quickly and you have no option but to endure it until you can leave or change the stimulation. In situations like this, remember that it is not your fault. It's no person's fault.

Caring for yourself in it all

Caregivers are known to have higher rates of depression, anxiety and burnout than other members of the community. Taking care of yourself means knowing and understanding yourself well enough to know your own signs of distress or 'early warning signs' that tell you that you need a break, a rest or time-out.

Monitoring for stress and agitation applies to you as well as to the person with dementia. What are your signs of distress? Notice your own signals that you need a break. There are support groups, people who can help to provide respite breaks, even for a couple of hours. Your self-awareness may be a work in progress as you become aware of how much you can tolerate, or how long you can keep up the constancy of caregiving before you start feeling you have a 'short fuse'. Plan breaks so you can avoid the disruptiveness and distress of burnout.

Feelings of guilt and thoughts of failure can plague you if you tend to blame yourself for needing to be cared for or to look after yourself. Some of us are not very good at it. If this is you, then you may need to talk to someone professionally who can help you work through your tendency to push away your own needs and struggle through. It may have helped you through life so far, but you will find it won't work with caregiving for someone with dementia.

Finally, there can be deep joy in caring for someone you love. In addition to the moments of struggle, grief and pain there can be hilarious moments that help to give you perspective. Play the long game of caregiving. This is a high mountain you are climbing with them and they will need you to the end.

Part II

A-Z OF DEMENTIA CARE AT HOME

Absconding

See *Unsafe leaving*

Abuse (in the past)

The person with dementia who you care for may have experienced abuse in their life. This may have been emotional, sexual, physical, mental, neglect, wartime or financial, or all/some of the above. Past abuse can lie dormant for decades until a moment occurs in which the person experiences a sensation (for example, image, smell, taste) similar to what they felt during the abuse. It may have been in childhood or adulthood. The earlier the abuse, the more difficult it may be to find a coherent narrative to explain it. Also, early abuse will have been influential on the formation of the person's sense of self. Early childhood abuse also has a profound effect on learning and development. It affects the ability to form trusting relationships, to relax with others, and let your guard down.

You may already know of the abuse when you commence your caregiving role or it may be revealed as time passes, or in a specific event. It can become obvious in the reactions of the person to personal care or your attempts to help, or when they make a mistake and anticipate punishment for it.

The onset of dementia can be the cause for activation of these well-defended past experiences. It can be as though the defensive

53

walls within the person begin to crack and become less solid. When they feel uncertain in dementia and unable to make sense of situations with the same confidence they developed as an adult, this can create a need to defend themselves, to prepare for criticism, assault or punishment, or to withdraw.

Watch for reactions that seem more intense or pronounced than you would normally expect. This will be further discussed in *Assault*, *Privacy* and *Trauma*.

Abuse (in the present)

See also *Assault*, *Safeguarding*

Abuse of elders is described by the World Health Organization as:

> an intentional act, or failure to act, by a caregiver or another person in a relationship involving an expectation of trust that causes harm to an adult 60 years and older... Abuse of older people can lead to serious physical injuries and long-term psychological consequences, increased risk of nursing home placement, use of emergency services, hospitalization and premature death. (World Health Organization, 2024)

As a caregiver, you need to be alert to the effect of your behaviour and words on the person you are caring for. We can be abusive without intending it. With the best of intentions, sometimes we can cause harm in our efforts to provide care. This may occur in attempting to assist a person with their hygiene, or it may be that we are abrupt and snappy in our speech to them repeatedly, so it becomes a habit. Others may notice it but we may not, unless we are alert to noticing our own behaviour.

Self-awareness and reflection on our own behaviour is a vital preventive of abusive behaviour as a caregiver.

You may come across people who engage in dominating, neglectful or intrusive behaviour towards those in their care. This is unacceptable and should be reported to police and safeguarding agencies.

Accusations

'You have stolen my purse.' 'You are keeping me prisoner.' Accusations can be made by a person with dementia about theft or the behaviour of caregivers towards them.

You may find that the person you care for makes accusations towards you about something you have or have not done. This can be very upsetting. You should take it seriously and adjust your behaviour so that the person you care for is respected and their preferences considered. For instance, if they accuse you of being a bully when you make them get dressed or showered in the mornings, consider how you could change your approach so that these negative feelings are not activated. It may be that you can be less direct and gentler, or use a reward to draw the person towards the behaviour you want rather than a commanding/instructing approach and tone. You may need to spend more time negotiating or perhaps model the behaviour you want. See Part I for a discussion of strategies to use.

If there is no foundation to the accusations it may be that the person with dementia has formed a belief that is not true. Try to investigate to make sure this is the case. Don't assume the person is making it up just because they have dementia. If you are a paid caregiver you should report to a family caregiver, if there is one, that the accusation has been made, and provide an account to your manager.

If you are a family member giving care for your spouse or parent, this is less clear, but it is sometimes useful to make sure someone else in the family knows what has occurred so that your own reputation in the family is protected. A shared approach can then be developed so that the false belief does not take root and become accepted as fact in the family or beyond.

If the accusation concerns someone else's behaviour, perhaps a paid caregiver or neighbour/friend, discuss it with the paid caregiver if possible. If this is not possible or does not resolve the issue and you continue to have concerns, you should report it to a manager and remain watchful for repetition, ready to protect the person you care for.

Activity

Activity is essential for physical, emotional, mental and social well-being. Being occupied is something we all take for granted until we can't participate or contribute as we may have in the past.

Each person will benefit from a tailored approach here. What I like to be active doing may not be your cup of tea. However, it is useful to think of the range of activities the person you care for is engaged in. Does it address each of the areas listed above? Is there enough physical activity? Is there sufficient mental stimulation to maintain skills for thinking, word-finding, problem-solving? Is it challenging enough, with ample opportunity for success?

Periods of activity and periods of rest throughout the day are important for balance. This rhythm provides interest and predictability. Having such a rhythm lowers stress levels and supports well-being. An example of such a rhythm is a sequence of the following: waking, breakfast, personal care, rest, a walk with the dog, return home for a cup of tea and biscuit, board game/cleaning/gardening, lunch. It's not complicated. It just requires a bit of thought and preparation. Think through the day and plan ahead.

Visit a social group or day centre where the person with dementia may engage with others in activities that are supported by paid professionals. Such activities may be a valuable source of skill maintenance and enjoyment. There are many benefits to such a connection. Regular attendance may provide something to look forward to and a way to punctuate the week.

In Australia, there are Planned Activity Groups (PAGs) which people with dementia may attend. These are government funded and designed to enhance the person's independence by promoting physical activity, cognitive stimulation, good nutrition, emotional well-being and social inclusion.[1] There are also day programmes that people living in their own homes may attend in a group. They return home at the end of the day having spent time with others in physical activity, social engagement, cognitive stimulation and sharing food. Check with your local agencies for similar organized day programmes.

---

1   www.dhhs.vic.gov.au

Adynamia

Adynamia is a condition that occurs when frontal lobe function of the brain is impaired, or a person is chronically depressed. It is characterized by lack of motivation and difficulty initiating actions. The person resists or finds reasons not to act, or is not interested. This can affect maintenance of functional skills.

For a caregiver, it can be frustrating to have to provide prompts to act, to do everyday tasks. However, without prompts the person may simply sit their day away, lose skills through lack of use and become further depressed.

To overcome adynamia, try breaking tasks into smaller parts so that each part is less onerous or looks less difficult, keeping a list of achievements, providing prompts for each part of the task, modelling the desired behaviour so the other person can mirror what they see you doing (see *Mirroring*).

Aggression

Aggression is often confused with anger. Anger is the emotion. Aggression is what we do or say. It is the action or words that communicate anger to others. The third element that is often mixed in here is violence. Violence is the use of physical force to injure, abuse or damage, usually in order to dominate another or inflict harm.

In dementia care, aggression most often consists of actions by the person with dementia to resist the actions of a caregiver. This most often occurs during personal care with activities such as dressing, showering or going to the toilet/bathroom. It may consist of hitting, pulling, grabbing, biting, pinching, kicking, and so on.

Two approaches need to be considered here: the first is preventative, the second is for 'after the horse has bolted'.

Preventative means thinking of how to avoid causing aggression in the first place and planning an approach that achieves a non-aggressive outcome. Think of aggression as the person's efforts to communicate their desire to be independent or to prevent themselves being overwhelmed by you. Try to look at it from their point of view. They are doing what they think is necessary to achieve their goal. So are you. You have the ability to step back and consider how to adjust your behaviour. They may not. So, it's up to you if the aggression is to change.

Aggression occurs when needs are not met or are frustrated. Tom Kitwood (1997) called this a state of ill-being. Needs not met means that we missed some cues that may have told us what the person prefers to be doing. By being aggressive the person is telling you something; for example, 'I'm not happy about what you are doing. I would prefer to be alone in my shower space like I always have been. You being here reminds me that I can't shower myself. Stop treating me like a child.'

First, identify the causes for aggression. It may be your behaviour, your tone or body language, or it may be the size of the bathroom, or the time of day, or that they wanted to sit in front of the television for longer, or the water is too hot or too cold, or the bathroom is too cold. Your assistance in getting them into the shower may make sense to you but it may be interpreted by them as dominating, intrusive and a downright nuisance. Think about your body language, the speed of your movements, the tone of your voice. Be careful not to adopt a patronizing tone. Be collegiate, a partner, an equal. Be slow in the speed of your movements so you don't hurry or hassle the person into moving too quickly, particularly during the undressing process. Take it step by step.

Talk if you know that that helps to maintain the connection, or be silent if you know talking agitates the person. Silent caregivers in residential care tend to be hit more often than caregivers who talk. Sometimes, a patter of what you have been up to or what you have planned or what friends have been doing can provide scaffolding for the person to relax and remain mentally connected with you during the showering process. It can also distract them from the physical process of showering or whatever you are engaged in doing together as they listen to you.

You can modify the causes. Make it pleasant and enjoyable. Put on some music they like, use a warm face-flannel like they do in Chinese restaurants and on some international flights, warm up the water, warm the towels, make it fun in whatever way you can. The person cannot be happy and angry at the same time.

The second approach is for after the aggression has occurred. Make yourself safe. Step back out of arm's reach. Then make the other person safe; in the shower scenario, turn the hot water off.

Ensure that no one is going to slip in water. Either stop the process of personal care and restart it when the mood has calmed, or move on to something else. Avoid shouting angrily but be very clear and direct in stating that this is not okay. 'You hit me. Stop it. Don't hit me' or 'You hit me. Stop it. Be gentle.' You may need to say both of these statements. One is negatively framed and the other is positively framed. Don't reward the undesirable behaviour with smiles and positive feedback. Make sure the message is that this is not okay. The person is the same behaviourally whether they are 8, 18 or 78.

Do not be blaming or make personal comments about them. Stay with the situation. Avoid saying 'You always...' or 'You never...' These statements are the bread and butter of marriage counselling.

Make sure you convey that this behaviour stops care. Step back, make yourself safe and stop bathing the person. If you have a hand-held shower, turn it away from the person and direct it at the wall of the shower space until the person calms. Your first statement can be as above: 'You hit me. Stop it. Don't hit me.' Then 'I can't shower you if you hit me.' Follow this up with the positively framed 'We can finish when you are calm.' The positive framing of the statement is important for directing the person's mind and attention towards the behaviour you want them to do. First, the limit setting ('Don't hit me. I can't shower you if you hit me') and then the positive framing to point the way forward. Resume only when they are calm. 'Okay. If you are feeling calm now we can start again. Can we start again?'

Using the *ABC model of behaviour* (see Part I), you can also utilize the consequences (C) to modify aggression. Aggression stops care, causes a breach in your emotional connection and creates aloneness. Aggression pushes people away from us. These are the natural consequences of aggression. It is not possible to be caring towards and emotionally available with someone who is aggressive. Nor is it possible to be connected and intimate with someone who is aggressive towards you. It is important to be clear about these natural consequences. Utilize them to help guide the person towards the behaviour you want more of by being consistent, clear and non-blaming.

Letting the person experience the natural consequences of their actions (within reasonable limits of physical and emotional safety) can help them to modify or control their own actions – step back and stop caregiving until they are calm and can participate in a non-aggressive manner.

Another approach is substitution (see Part I). You can have the person hold a soft sponge, if they are able, so they can contribute to the showering process and so they have a soft object in their hands when they go to hit you. You may have a wet face but it hurts less than a fist or open hand. The same 'step back, stop care' sequence should then be followed.

Agitation

Agitation is the behavioural sign of a disturbed internal state. The person is not at peace, nor contented. You will see pacing, facial grimace, hand and arm movements, touching the face repeatedly, repetitive questioning, sweating, aggressive outbursts, tearfulness, clinging, seeking, restlessness.

It can be activated by time of day (see *Sundowning*), an event, hunger, thirst, or illness and pain. A diagnostic approach is useful here. The first step is to eliminate possible physical causes. Is there illness or pain? Is there hunger or thirst? Then explore emotional upset. Has an event occurred such as someone visiting or an interaction at day care that upset the person and is still upsetting them hours later? Then explore environmental causes: is it the time of day? For instance, has this occurred in a pattern that indicates that between 4 and 5pm the person begins pacing and looking for home?

It may be that a medical assessment is necessary to eliminate physical causes. If the person has a urinary tract infection they can become agitated as a result of the infection. Prompt treatment with antibiotics is required to address this and return the person to health.

Pain is a common cause of agitation. It may not be possible for the person to tell you they have pain, or to describe it. You will have to rely on what you can see and hear in order to connect the dots as it were. See *Pain*.

Agnosia

This is a brain problem that means the person is unable to recognize objects that were previously familiar. It is relatively common as dementia progresses. They can see the objects but not recognize them. They do not understand how to use them or interact with them. This may affect personal activities of daily living such as dressing, because the person may not recognize clothing and not know what to do with it. It may also affect eating as they do not recognize food or utensils and are not able to eat independently.

If this occurs it is not usually helpful to point out to the person that they have failed to recognize an object as this risks them becoming upset and resentful about their mistake and you pointing it out. It is better to simply and quietly provide the assistance required to bridge the missing ability. For example, when dressing, lift up the piece of clothing and hold it in front of the person. Offer it to them and say, 'This is your shirt, put your arm in here.' See *Dressing* and *Eating*.

Agnosia may also affect recognition of faces and voices. This can be very upsetting for family members as they realize that Mum or Dad or their friend no longer recognizes them or only intermittently recognizes them. If this occurs, it is best to not point it out but for them to introduce themselves to the person with dementia and commence a conversation that can cause recognition by activating memory for past events. Acting in a familiar manner may help the person with dementia to access who the other person is in another way. If the face doesn't do it, the voice might. Perhaps singing together may cause recognition.

Other senses can also be involved. This may include smells such as previously liked perfumes, scents or aromas. Food that was valued and usually caused the person to come into the kitchen and look forward to the meal may no longer trigger this response. However, it may still draw the person into the kitchen where they may wonder what they came in for.

Agnosia can lead to other people pulling away as they sense that the person with dementia no longer recognizes them. Friends no longer call in. Adult children may come round less frequently and relate to the person with dementia through the caregiver in phone calls rather than face-to-face visits. This increased social isolation can be toxic for the person and is to be avoided if possible by encouraging family and friends to maintain their visits and activities for as long as possible. Offer them ways to have a visit. See *Visiting*.

Alcohol

Alcohol does not help brain function. It is a central nervous system depressant that reduces mental function and responsiveness to the world around us. It also dulls our awareness of internal experience, which is often why we use it – to reduce a sense of tension inside which we equate with being relaxed. It also has a disinhibiting effect, so we feel freer to act without social constraints. An example of disinhibited behaviour is loud talking, swearing, or being more affectionate or aggressive when intoxicated.

That said, a beer or glass of wine as a regular part of life can be a source of enjoyment, particularly if it is a habit and something you both do together. Stopping it may be counterproductive. More than one glass may not be helpful as the disinhibition caused by alcohol may lead to reduced ability to stop angry urges or reduced problem-solving ability. It may also affect social awareness and lead to antisocial behaviour.

Alcohol abuse and withdrawal can cause delirium and should be controlled to avoid the negative effect on mental function.

All-or-nothing thinking

See also *Cognitive distortions*

This is a type of cognitive distortion that influences thinking and behaviour so that we think in extremes without including the wide range of possibilities. It is also known as 'black-and-white' thinking, and either/or thinking. There are no shades of grey in this style of thinking. Examples include: He is always... He is never... People are good or bad, lazy or hard-working, lovable or detestable. One's actions can be successful or an abject failure. A person who thinks this way can flip between extremes in their attitude to you.

It is a pattern of thinking that causes instability and extremes of emotional reaction that follow changes in thinking from one pole to another. Mood swings can be extreme.

See *Black-and-white thinking*.

Alzheimer's disease

This disease was first described by Alois Alzheimer in 1906 when he noticed changes in the brain tissue of Auguste D. who died following memory loss, language problems and abnormal behaviour. From the autopsy, he noticed that the patient's brain had decreased in size. Alzheimer's disease now accounts for 60–70 per cent of dementia diagnoses.

Subsequently, research has identified proteins including beta-amyloid and tau associated with Alzheimer's disease. Despite a great deal of research effort, the mechanisms underlying Alzheimer's disease are not fully understood.

Several medications have been developed to modify the symptoms of memory loss and agitation and slow the progress of the disease. See also *Dementia*.

Announcing care

This is a communication technique in which a caregiver provides notice of their intention to provide care prior to commencing the care activity: 'Darling, I am about to start the shower for you.' This activates the brain to be ready to respond.

The benefits of announcing care include keeping stress low by avoiding startling the person, and giving the person with dementia an opportunity to respond, indicating cooperation or refusal. This prevents a potential conflict and maintains your relationship in a positive mode.

Annoyed

Annoyed, irritated, frustrated, angry. These are all synonyms for anger, perhaps of varying degrees. Annoyance is an internal state of emotion that is characterized by an increase in arousal and readiness to act.

Antecedent

Anything that comes before another thing is an antecedent. In dementia care, this term is often used to describe the factors that influence or cause a behaviour. It is commonly used in the *ABC model of behaviour* (see Part I).

Anti-anxiety medication

The most common anti-anxiety medications are benzodiazepines. Benzodiazepines are *not recommended* for the treatment of agitation and anxiety in dementia care. They have been associated with higher rates of dependence, mobility problems, confusion, sedation and mortality in the elderly. Anti-anxiety drugs have in the past been frequently used as an initial response to behavioural problems in dementia care.

They have different common names in each country. This class of drug includes: Diazepam (Valium), Temazepam (Temaze, Normison), Oxazepam (Serepax, Serax, Alepam), Lorazepam (Ativan, Lorazepam Intensol, Loreev XR) and Clonazepam (Klonopin).

If the person you care for has intolerable anxiety you should first engage with psychological and medical assessment and advice. If the medical opinion is to use benzodiazepines as a first step, ensure that it will usually be for short-term relief only and monitoring for confusion/sedation and balance and mobility problems. Ensure that the response includes exploration of a range of reasons for the person's anxiety (see *Medication, Anxiety*).

Antidepressant medication

Drugs that are used to treat depression are known as antidepressants. They are also used to treat anxiety, obsessive compulsive disorder (OCD) and post-traumatic stress disorder (PTSD). The list of antidepressants in common use is long. The most common group of antidepressants is selective serotonin reuptake inhibitors (SSRIs). These work by altering the amount of serotonin available in the brain so that the person's mood is improved and their anxiety is decreased. Information on antidepressants is widely available.

In dementia care, antidepressants have been found to have variable effects. Some people respond well but others do not.

Antipsychotic medication

Antipsychotic medication is not recommended for people with dementia due to increased mortality and cardiac problems. However, some antipsychotic medications are used 'off-label' by prescribers to manage behavioural disturbance.

Medication for psychosis has evolved in recent decades. In the past, drugs used for psychosis were often used long term and had terrible side-effects that reduced quality of life and often caused permanent problems such as tardive dyskinesia (a condition where your face, body or both make sudden, irregular movements).

Recent developments in antipsychotic drugs have seen improvements so that such effects are rarely seen these days. The side-effects are fewer and the prescribing approach is usually to start low and go slow.

Anxiety

Anxiety is the human experience of response to risk or threat. It is most frequently experienced as panic, fear, stress, tension. It involves activation of the central nervous system to cause a person to protect themselves by fleeing or fighting or freezing, depending on the nature and severity of the threat. Anxiety appears to have an evolutionary purpose of improving survival.

Anxiety achieves this by releasing adrenalin from the adrenal glands that sit on top of the kidneys. This flushes into the bloodstream causing tightening of muscles in readiness for action, and increased heart rate to improve blood supply to the muscles. Digestion stops and the desire to urinate increases as the person becomes focused solely on responding to threat. Thinking becomes focused on the source of threat, and scanning for threat becomes a mental priority.

All of this is fine if you have a mammoth descending on you. However, if you live in a place where there are few mammoths and the risks of physical attack are minimal, such an experience will be an unpleasant interruption to your otherwise calm life. But this is the lot of many people who live with chronic anxiety.

For people living with dementia, anxiety is increased largely due to the effects of memory loss, difficulties with thinking and solving problems, and the increased frequency of mistakes. This leads to insecurity and uncertainty, negative self-talk and recriminations on the part of the person with dementia as they contend with changes in their ability to perform tasks at which they were previously successful.

Anxiety in dementia is also a product of the insecurity about who they are now and where they belong or fit in. Am I still valuable and lovable, worthwhile? Am I safe, protected and secure? Do I really belong anymore? Am I a burden? These are fundamental fears that sit within us until a crisis flushes them to the surface of our minds.

Once anxious, we find ourselves living with it, thinking that anxiety is necessary to keep us safe, worthwhile or belonging: 'I must keep ruminating [going over and over it] so I can successfully prevent myself making that same mistake again. That way I will be safe from criticism and won't feel bad and I won't be rejected as a failure.' So being anxious can be seen by the anxious person as a good thing. They cannot live without it and do not want to give it up.

The pity of it is that this ruminating/worrying/panicking/obsessing/stressing prevents us from concentrating on what is actually happening around us and causes us to make more mistakes and live with poorer quality of life. It makes us more uncertain and preoccupied with anxiety itself. So we become anxious about being anxious.

For a person living with dementia, anxiety can be an unwelcome companion. Old anxieties surface and preoccupations that were long forgotten can re-emerge to plague the person with uncertainty and distress. Hard-won confidence in adulthood can disappear in the face of small errors or repeated forgetting. Childhood insecurity surfaces.

Management of anxiety in dementia can include reassurance that the person is safe, removing whatever is provoking the anxiety, or removing the person from it (for example, go home from the shopping centre), using a calm voice and diverting the person to another focus until they calm down. Avoid denying that they have any reason for being anxious. This invalidates the person and may result in them withdrawing or escalating the anxious response.

Apathy

Lack of interest, enthusiasm or concern, indifference – this definition is an apt description of apathy in dementia. It is common for people with dementia to experience apathy at times. They may be difficult to motivate to get dressed, leave the house or take a shower. Apathy places a burden on the caregiver to provide the motivation or at least to coax the person to engage in the activity. In research, apathy has been associated with nursing home placement, caregiver distress, and decreased well-being for the person with dementia.

If apathy is due to frontal lobe impairment, it may require medication, combined with identifying the person's needs for comfort, relationship, occupation, inclusion. Although they may not have a 'felt' experience of the need themselves, they will give signals of discomfort or irritation if their needs are not met. By knowing these signals, the caregiver can provide comfort and activity in a timely way that maintains the person in a positive state.

Art

Dementia can be an opportunity for new engagement in artistic expression. Creativity stays with a person with dementia well into the progression of the underlying condition. This may take the form of painting or drawing, of playing in an imaginative way, dance or body movement, song/vocalizing, listening to or making music, making objects with media such as clay, wood, and so on. The list is endless. It is important to not limit the creativity to conventional forms of artistic expression. Rather, as a caregiver, provide the person with opportunities to engage with the materials for creation, then see what they want to do.

You may find that they can engage in artistic expression only if they can see someone else doing it around them. This is a common phenomenon in dementia care. If they can see it, they can do it.

> A daughter noticed that her mother did not knit anymore unless she was sitting with someone else who knitted.

Support or scaffolding is crucial for people with dementia. The presence of someone else doing the same activity acts as a form of scaffolding that can not only prompt the person to engage in it but can support or carry them into and through the activity.

It is important to know how much scaffolding to provide and when. Too much and the person will be overwhelmed and stop; too little and they will become discouraged and stop. Too soon and they will not get the chance to use their skills and residual knowledge; too late and they will give up in frustration.

Provide the materials, the set-up and the supportive presence and the person with dementia may be able to experience successful artistic creativity and hence improve their well-being.

Success is not the production of a piece of art. Success is whatever the person with dementia regards as success. So as a caregiver, be focused on their signals of well-being, interest and concentration. This means monitoring and perhaps withholding your comments or feedback that can shape the other person's sense of how they are going. Avoid corrective comments unless physical safety is at stake. Your comments should be enough to maintain the person's activity but not go over the top or lead them to do what you think is good or worthwhile. Let the person with dementia guide your actions and words in this interaction. It is for their benefit, not yours.

Assault

You may notice during personal care that the person with dementia reacts strongly to being touched. It may be fearful, or aggressive. This is often evidence of previous experiences of being assaulted which may be in recent times or in the distant past. If you suspect it is in recent times you should report your experiences.

If it is more likely to be have been in the distant past (that is, there have been no other caregivers), you may need to adjust your personal care assistance so they can lower their fear or aggression response and you can build or rebuild trust.

Be clear in your verbal and non-verbal communication that you mean no harm, that you are there to help, that they can choose what they want help with or when or how much help they want. Smile, remind them who you are if they have forgotten. Keep up a continual stream of talk or chatter. Caregivers who go silent are more likely to be assaulted themselves as the person loses connection with them and is then unable to make sense of why this person is in their private space touching them. Be clear to the person with dementia that they have power to influence the way care is provided. There may be some non-negotiables such as hygiene and emotional well-being. These are outcomes. How you get there is not as important as the goals.

See also *Abuse, Trauma*.

Assertiveness

Assertiveness is when we meet our own needs without dominating or becoming aggressive in speech or actions. It sits between compliance and dominance. You may find that the person with dementia becomes more or less assertive.

Assertiveness is usually healthy because the person does or says something to meet their own needs. It may come as a surprise if we are not accustomed to seeing the person asserting themselves. It may take the form of stating an opinion about food: 'I don't like that.' Or perhaps about timing of personal care: 'I want to go now' or, 'Don't do it that way.'

Simply accept the assertive statement: 'Okay, thanks for telling me. What about trying this?' If you accept, the person's communication will often lead to them settling or at least remaining in a calm state without them needing to say it again.

Avoid arguing. This can escalate the level of aggression and there is usually only one winner in such a contest.

Assisting

Assisting is a way of helping a person with dementia by supplying what they cannot do for themselves independently. It means *doing with* the person rather than *doing for* the person. For example, with mealtimes, only provide what the person cannot do for themselves. In personal care, you might place clothing out on the bed if you know they cannot find or sort objects easily but can put them on once objects are placed in the right order for them. Do not take over and do it for them, which might be quicker and tidier but could rob them of their skills.

LIVING WITH A PERSON WITH DEMENTIA

Assisting is like scaffolding. It supports the person to be successful, and in the end it becomes invisible and only the building remains.

Brain skills require regular use to remain intact. Use it or lose it. By assisting the person, we help them have success and so maintain their self-esteem and self-agency. We also help their brain to stay active and working effectively for as long as possible.

See *Mealtimes, Eating, Feeding, Person-centred care.*

Attachment

See Part I for an extensive discussion of attachment.

Attention

Attention is the brain's ability to focus, to maintain awareness of the world around you, and the world inside you.

If something interests you or someone asks you a question, you pay attention. You give them your attention. Mostly, you focus attention automatically, so you take it for granted. You listen without having to consciously work at it. And if it becomes boring you lose attention and drift off in a daydream.

Attention is vital for communication and remembering. It can be impaired by dementia. The person with dementia may have trouble paying attention to what you say. This may be more of a problem as memory loss progresses – if they have difficulty paying attention they may also have trouble remembering information.

If as a carer you need a person with dementia to take notice of something you say, you must ensure that you have their attention. The best way to get a person's attention is to have them look at you. Make eye contact with them, then say what you want them to take in. Reduce distracting sources of noise such as music or television.

Attention-seeking

Seeking attention is sometimes seen as a negative: 'He's just attention-seeking.' However, attention is what makes your social survival possible. Without it you can shrivel up and die, or become depressed and withdraw.

The term 'attention-seeking' is a problem in itself and I would encourage you to avoid it. Find some other words to describe what the person is doing. If someone is seeking attention there will be a good reason for it. If they want your attention, consider yourself privileged to be the person they want to have connection with.

You have to first understand the reason and then you can respond appropriately to meet the need that is driving the attention-seeking behaviour. It always happens for a reason. The act of wanting attention from you is an expression of an inner unmet need for recognition, acknowledgement or connection. It may be that in their early life they were not the apple of anyone's eye, they were not the focus of their parents' attention and never received the recognition or acknowledgement that they even existed as a feeling being. Many children grew up unrecognized as anything other than an extension of their parents and objects to be controlled and managed. Or perhaps they always had someone's attention and did not develop the capacity to be by themselves and be motivated by their own desires. When dementia occurs and the inner controls on their own behaviour decrease, these unmet needs can emerge.

You may find that the need for attention is deeply felt and nothing you do can satisfy it. In this case, in the short term you may need to distract the person to something more appealing and then be proactive with recognition, acknowledgement or connection, without waiting for the need to be felt and the attention-seeking behaviour to emerge. Proactively provide what is missing in the person with dementia, and they will be more content and settled. This will take practice and repetition.

Back off

Backing off is what you do when you need to decrease the pressure on the other person to avoid making the situation worse.

It may mean physically removing yourself if it is safe to do so. If it is not safe to do so, backing off may simply be that you stop talking. Or talk more quietly or slowly. Or it may be that you smile and say, 'Oh well, we don't have to go if you don't want to', or, 'No problem, we can leave that till tomorrow if you like.'

It is a judicious withdrawal aimed at relieving tension and an

LIVING WITH A PERSON WITH DEMENTIA

escalation in feelings that you sense could lead to an explosion. Backing off allows the person with dementia to return to a calm state.

It also avoids dominating the person into submission. This is always a bad thing because it results in the person being the loser in a battle. Avoid at all costs. They are losing enough without your need to win being the cause of another loss. Again, if physical safety is at stake you will need to develop the ability to distract them to something else and soothe the situation. Move on to something more attractive that involves less confrontation.

> Robert sees that it is raining as Eve puts on her coat and makes ready to go for her regular walk. He points out the rain and she becomes annoyed, accusing him of being negative and wanting to stop her all the time. Robert quietly replies, 'Well, we could always go into town to the cinema. What do you think?' This appeals to Eve as he knows she relishes the cosiness of the cinema and the early days of their relationship sitting together in the darkness of the back row. She settles and they begin preparations to go into town.

An alternative ending may have been:

> Robert replies, 'Okay, go for a walk if you like. I'll be here when you get back with a towel and some dry clothes.' Eve goes outside but is back in a few minutes having become very wet from the rain. She announces, 'It's raining. I'm not going out in that.'

Sometimes if physical safety is not at stake it may be best to allow the situation to unfold and resolve. More often than not, nothing bad will happen and the consequences will not be dire, permanent or dangerous. And the person with dementia gets to exercise agency and experience the satisfaction of success.

Bathing

This private activity is essential for hygiene and personal presentation. It is usually something you do daily, in private with your own routines that prepare you for the day and who you will meet.

Hygiene, dignity, identity and *well-being* are the outcomes. You have routines and rituals that you go through, which may evolve over time but which usually you perform competently on your own.

However, when dementia comes along, bathing, whether it is using the toilet, taking a bath or showering, shaving, or putting makeup on, these well-practised activities can become complicated and difficult. Memory and sequencing problems may interfere with the fluent step-wise processes that previously got the person with dementia from nightwear to fully dressed and groomed.

This usually means you will be called on to assist. This is known as personal care. The assistance you need to provide will change over time as the person's needs change. Imagine a sliding scale of caregiving. On one end is no assistance and on the other end is full assistance. As dementia progresses and impairments increase, the slide moves from one end to the other. Depending on the situation, it may move back and forwards. It is important to be flexible and adapt your caregiving to what is needed to ensure the person is successful.

Try to ensure that the person does as much as they can for themselves. It can be tempting to take over and prevent moments of uncertainty or error. However, it is better to wait and be there to provide the bridging comment that enables them to move across to the next part of the task as independently as possible. Independence is important for brain health. The person's brain has to work when they are independent. When they are dependent on you, your brain is doing the work and theirs gets a holiday.

A couple of practical tips may help here. Ensure that the bathroom is comfortable and items are where the person can see them. You may need to modify the bathroom cabinet so that all items can be seen. This overcomes forgetting where things are. If you don't want the person having access to some items all the time due to them squeezing the toothpaste every time they see it, you may have to put it out only when it is needed and have a safety-access device on the bathroom cabinet.

Warm up the towels in the clothes dryer for a few minutes prior to a bath so the experience is as pleasant as possible. Make sure the temperature of the room is comfortable.

See also *Toilet, Privacy, Assault, Abuse, Trauma.*

Bedwetting

Wetting the bed at night can occur when dementia affects the involuntary muscles that you rely on as an adult to ensure you remain continent. Practically you can prepare for such an event by ensuring that the bed has a waterproof cover over the mattress and under the linen. Have ready a change of pyjamas.

Night-time *incontinence* can be very distressing for anyone. However, it can be particularly distressing for a person with dementia, who may be unable to understand the discomforting sensations of wetness they have experienced. Even if they cannot make full sense of it, at some depth they may know they have done something that they shouldn't have done.

Alternatively, they may be very aware of what has happened and feel ashamed and angry with themselves. Your response will determine how deeply embarrassed they feel or not.

With an eye on their feelings, it is best to remain gently focused on the series of tasks to return the person to bed: remove their clothing, wash or shower, re-dress and comfort them, change the bed linen and return the person to bed in a calm state.

They may be unable to make sense of what has happened. If they are confused by it you may be able to engage them in conversation that has nothing to do with bedwetting but which you know is something they can participate in readily. If you can engage them with music or an activity, you can go about washing them, changing the bed, and so on.

See also *Soiling, Incontinence, Continence*.

Behaviour

Behaviour is what you do or say. Any action that is observable by others is behaviour. Behaviour communicates your inner experience to others and theirs to you. Any time you do or say anything, you are behaving. So in its simplest meaning, it is not about good behaviour or bad behaviour, it's just behaviour – what you can see or hear.

Behaviour is the 'B' in the *ABC model of behaviour management*: Antecedent, Behaviour and Consequence. This is an old model of behaviour and is oversimplified and misused. However, the benefit of it is that it gets across the idea that behaviour occurs for a reason and that there are consequences. There is always a cause or reason, an antecedent that comes before the behaviour. And there are always consequences.

If you can identify the cause, you can often work out what the response should be to meet the need that drives the behaviour in the first place. In a person-centred approach, remember that behaviour always occurs in a situation, in a person with a history, with a personality, with social preferences, with a physical and medical history, all of which contribute to cause a behaviour to be stimulated. It is often not just one cause.

The cause is most often unmet needs in the person. They communicate to you their unmet needs in their behaviour. If you treat behaviour as a message, a communication, you will live with fewer control battles and a more content person.

See *Causes, behavioural, Consequences.*

Behaviour Support Team

This is a multidisciplinary team that provides support to people caring for anyone living with dementia at home or in long-term residential care. They provide assessment and ongoing support functions, with ideas and practical knowledge to assist you in providing care for a person with dementia. These teams exist in most countries and are funded variously through donations or by government. What they do will vary from country to country. Your local Alzheimer's dementia organization is a good place to start for further information. You can also find out more by doing an online search for 'dementia behaviour support' or similar.

Behavioural consequences

This is an approach to the management of behaviour that I do not recommend is used with anyone with dementia. It is a term that is used frequently in everyday speech, but it is a problem when applied to people living with dementia. I will first explain what it is and then why it should not be used, except in certain situations.

Behavioural consequences is the use of consequences to encourage or discourage behaviour. It involves a person choosing to do or avoid a behaviour once it is pointed out to them. It is delivered with a two-part statement to the person so they can remember it when the situation happens again. For example: 'If... then...'

Examples to illustrate: If you go out on the road then you could be run over by a car. If you don't lift your feet, you will trip over. If you have a drink late at night, you might wet the bed. If you walk out in the rain, you will get wet. If you don't have a shower, you will smell bad around other people. If you shout at me, I can't hear you.

This approach relies on memory. The person has to have a capacity to remember what you said earlier when the situation occurs next. It also requires a form of associative thinking that is rather too complex for many people with dementia. It also asks that the person with dementia engages in abstract thinking, which may be too difficult for them. They have to think about a future situation that is not yet happening.

That said, it may be that you can use this in a simple form in the immediate situation such as preparing for shopping: 'If you don't get dressed in your good clothes, we won't be able to go shopping.' You could rephrase it into a positive statement: 'If you get dressed in your good clothes, we can go shopping.' Work out what you and the person you care for can manage and work with that. Keep it positive and use it in the present moment. Don't use it where it relies on them to remember the link you made (If... then...) from one mealtime to the next or one day to the next. Keep it concrete, specific and immediate. Dressing in good clothes to go shopping *now*.

Bereavement

The death of people close to us causes sadness and a sense of loss. It can also cause an awareness of our own mortality and the brief nature of our own existence.

Bereavement is the normal and expected reaction to loss. You grieve in proportion to the depth/intensity of the love and bond you feel for the person/animal/object/role you have lost.

Psychiatrist and author Elizabeth Kübler-Ross proposed five stages in the grieving process: denial, anger, bargaining, depression and acceptance. Whether these stages describe your experience or not they can be a guide to being patient with yourself and others who are taking some time to come to grips with losing someone close to them.

Death is not the only reason for bereavement. There is grief in the losses that occur on a daily basis in dementia care. As the person with dementia loses abilities, and changes before your eyes, you will likely experience grief for the person you knew and loved. This repeated loss has been described as a daily death, and an ongoing funeral.

Respect your own grief, and allow yourself to feel the sadness and anger that come with having a person you love taken from you. But also allow yourself to feel the love with the sadness and anger. This mix of feelings can feel intolerable at times, but if you didn't feel love, you wouldn't be sad and angry. It is a core part of loving that we will feel sadness and anger.

Black-and-white thinking

See *All-or-nothing thinking*

Boredom

Most of us become bored at some point in our lives. Boredom is what you experience when you have little or no stimulation. It is unpleasant to be bored. If it goes on for long enough you may go to sleep, or alternatively you may find something to fill the vacuum. *Occupation* is a fundamental need. Without it you can slip into *depression*. Your brain does not like being bored and will seek out sleep or activity and stimulation to relieve it. Usually, you will be able to find something to relieve the boredom and stimulate your interest.

In dementia, the person may have a reduced capacity due to memory loss or other processing limitations, or they may have reduced opportunities for stimulation. Just because the person has dementia doesn't mean they cannot think or remember or desire something. People with dementia need activity (not all the time of course, but in a rhythm of activity and rest). They are no different from you and me.

To relieve boredom, the person with dementia may find something to do of interest and it may be inconvenient for others or it may be unsafe. If you don't want the person to be bored and find their own solution, you may have to provide regular input or opportunities for stimulation that they find satisfying.

See *Activity*.

Boundaries

As a caregiver, you will be called on to be ready to assist, provide bridging, scaffold the other person's life and help them get through the minor and major moments of crisis that occur. Through it all you may lose contact with your friends and your extended family. You may find it consumes you.

You will need to have boundaries that enable you to take time for yourself. This is important to avoid the exhaustion and depression of burnout. Your boundaries enable you to say, 'No, I can't be there that day.' To do this you will need to plan ahead and organize someone else to replace you. It may be a respite service which provides someone to give you a break. Check with your local services.

Brain

The brain is one of our organs required for survival. It enables us to think, feel, remember, process sensory information, perceive the world and respond to it. It is composed of two hemispheres and several lobes or sections, with specific areas associated with functions (for example, the temporal lobes are associated with memory and emotional processing). There is an area for language production and another for language comprehension.

There has been a significant growth in knowledge and understanding of brain function in the past couple of decades. Brain scans and electron microscopes have allowed us to see what has previously been a mystery to scientists. Neurons, glia and proteins all function to produce thought and mind. It has been said that mind is what the brain does.

The brain has the capacity to renew, to produce new neurons continually through life. Neuroplasticity is a relatively new phenomenon to us. However, the brain has always been able to change, to adapt to changes, to injuries. Now we are beginning to understand better how to work with the brain to make the most of its capacity to adapt, to learn, to change.

See *Brain cells*.

Brain cells

Neurons are the basic building blocks of the brain. They are a type of nerve cell that allows the brain to function. They work by making chemical and electrical impulses that send 'messages' from one neuron to another. Like a tree has roots, trunk and branches, neurons have connections to other neurons. These connections tell the next neuron to turn on or off. There are several types of neurons, each located in a specific area of the brain, depending on their function. Neurons rely on a fine balance of chemicals and nutrients provided by the glial cells.

It is believed that Alzheimer's disease is caused by plaques and tangles that cause a malfunction of neurons. Plaques and tangles are proteins in the brain that occur in abnormal amounts and malfunction to interfere with normal brain function. They are found in high levels in the brains of people with Alzheimer's disease.

The other type of brain cells is glia. They are located throughout the brain. Their main function is to support the work of the neurons. They outnumber neurons and act as scavengers, as stimulators of neurons, and they communicate with neurons.

Burnout

Burnout is a state of mental, physical and emotional exhaustion and is the consequence of severe and prolonged stress. It is common in the workplace and in caregiving roles where people are exposed to prolonged stress that feels inescapable. People can lose hope and feel trapped, as if the demands are endless and resources are diminishing.

Signs of burnout include exhaustion, a sense of emptiness, difficulty sleeping, fatigue, negative outlook and sense of hopelessness, becoming irritable, fearful, cynical and impatient, difficulty concentrating, and reduced sense of personal accomplishment.

Risk factors for burnout include low self-esteem, lack of

control over workload, not knowing how to cope, unrealistically high expectations, conflict and effort-reward imbalance. Chronic burnout can result in post-traumatic stress if conditions are not addressed.

Prevention or treatment can include ensuring that you have support that you can trust to provide the resources you need as conditions change. This requires you to reach out to others, let others know what you need in time to provide it before a crisis develops. Exercise regularly. Eat well. Be flexible and realistic in your expectations. If, as a carer, you find that you are not flexible or your expectations are proving unrealistic, get some help to address this professionally and early so that it does not build to a crisis in which the person with dementia cannot stay at home any longer.

Caregiving

Caregiving is the practical and emotional experience of providing support and assistance to another who is in need. We do it to ensure we survive as a species. It feels good to care for another person in need.

Caregiving has traditionally been regarded as a female activity. Up to 95 per cent of paid caregivers are female and there are cultural and historical reasons for this. However, we know that males can provide care as well. Caregiving is not a gendered activity. Anyone can do it. An increasing number of males are entering the paid caregiving workforce and this is slowly changing.

Dementia caring involves practical actions of helping a person to eat, dress, bathe, go to the toilet, socialize, relax and play, shop, and so on. In other words, you enable the person to be successful at everyday activities. In person-centred caring, it means only providing what the person cannot do for themselves, and not doing everything for them. See *Person-centred care*.

It also is an emotional experience of feeling warmth and regard for the person you care for. These positive emotions draw you towards the person so you can comfort and connect with them when they suffer or experience distress.

Catastrophizing

This pattern of thinking is characterized by assuming the worst. You can live as though disaster is always about to befall you. You can live with a sense of dread, negativity and hopelessness that the inevitable failure and doom is about to occur.

In dementia, this can take the form of a tendency to hopelessness, and feelings of despair in the face of mistakes that may occur.

Causes, behavioural

Causes of behaviour are discussed in detail in Part I.

Celebration

There will be moments in your caregiving relationship with a person with dementia that are important to celebrate. Celebration is the act of making a moment significant, marking an event so it stands out, and rewarding a positive achievement or success.

Birthdays, anniversaries or just a regular weekly meal can be moments for celebration. Equally, and perhaps more important, are those everyday moments when someone with dementia achieves something they usually cannot do. By celebrating their success, we mark it as a positive experience and signal to them that this is important and valuable.

The fact that they remembered to dress for the weather may be cause for a positive comment. The celebration does not have to be streamers and whistles. Rather, it can be a quiet affirmation of success in a gentle positive comment or a smile of acknowledgement that says, 'I see you. I understand how important that was for you.'

Challenging behaviour

This is a term used to describe behaviour that you find difficult. It usually includes aggression, demanding, shouting/yelling, escaping, hitting, and so on. Other terms for this type of behaviour include *disturbed behaviour* and *disruptive behaviour*. Usually, the focus is on the effect of the behaviour on others, if it is challenging or disturbing or disruptive for others. Terms such as these have been the subject of much discussion among clinicians in recent decades as perceptions of this behaviour have changed.

The principal problem with this term is that it ignores the person, treats them as the problem and makes no attempt to understand why the behaviour occurred. It also treats the behaviour as though it occurs in a vacuum.

A focus on the effect of the behaviour on others has led to a 'management' approach. The emphasis historically has been on controlling the social effect on other people. People who behave in this manner were and still are separated from mainstream society and admitted to hospitals where they were/are treated as patients with an illness or housed in institutions.

A more healthy and reasonable approach to this behaviour is to understand it as dementia *distress behaviour*.

Choices

Enabling a person to make choices supports their abilities, empowers and enhances their personhood. Making choices makes your brain work. The more it works, the more it remains functional. Use it or lose it.

Offering a choice to someone is an everyday activity that we do with each other in the normal flow of the day. 'What would you like for lunch?'

When it comes to someone with dementia, choices are important for making their brain work and for sending a message that they remain a participating person in their relationship with you. Choices give you power to influence your world.

Being offered a choice gives the person the opportunity to remain a functioning equal in the social world. Choices are vital for mental and emotional health.

Choices must be offered for success. If their ability to consider an open question, such as 'What would you like for lunch?', is impaired, make the offering into a yes/no question: 'Would you like a ham sandwich?' Adjust your offering to what they can succeed with.

Sometimes you may find that a judicious suggestion can simplify a complex array of options into something more manageable. For instance, if the person is dressing for an outing and they are confronted with multiple shirts to choose from, a comment such as 'That check shirt looks good on you' may simplify the options and make the choice manageable.

Church

See also *Religion, Faith, Spirituality*

The practice of religious faith may provide a person with dementia with comfort and meaning. The rituals of church attendance and participation in worship are familiar routines that can enable a person with dementia to continue participating with ease and comfort.

As dementia progresses, the extent of their participation may need to be adjusted. A person who has taken communion all their life may find at some point in the progress of their condition that they become confused by the object that is placed on their palm or tongue and uncertain about what to do with it. Being by their shoulder can make this moment smooth, with a quiet suggestion as to what to do with it. You may need to help them adjust their participation over time so it remains a positive and enhancing experience.

Church attendance can be an opportunity to educate the church community about dementia and help them to be more comfortable, inclusive and supportive.

Closeness

See also *Attachment*

Closeness refers to emotional closeness. Depending on the nature of your relationship with the person who has dementia, it may be an emotionally close, neutral or emotionally distant relationship. Their past experience will usually indicate the amount of emotional intimacy they are comfortable with.

For some people, being emotionally close is tremendously important and a regular part of each day. For others, emotional closeness can be a source of anxiety and stress and cause them to put emotional and/or physical distance between themselves and others, including you.

The level of comfort with emotional closeness has a lot to do with early life experiences of attachment. Some people with a secure attachment story will be more comfortable with emotional closeness and secure with distance. Others who have an insecure story of early attachment may be anxious about being alone and demanding of your presence. This can be constant as their anxiety seems bottomless. Others again may be content with emotional distance and not require much comforting and actually be stressed if you want to be too close or around them all the time.

It is important to think about why they might be wanting or avoiding closeness, so you can understand it and manage your own reactions, because your own attachment history will shape your reactions to being held at a distance or followed around all day.

If you are naturally avoidant of closeness you may find it stressful to have someone follow you or want to be near you or even hold your hand. It may be that your priority is a clean and well-ordered house rather than building trust and participation. If you understand where this is coming from in yourself you may be able to manage it without pushing the other person away and making them secondary to your efficiency.

If, on the other hand, you naturally want closeness and the other person is avoidant, you become resentful of their distance given all you do for them. If they are also wanting closeness, you may find it necessary to create some boundaries or limits that allow you to do the practical things that need to be done around the house or with the person with dementia.

Cognitive behavioural therapy (CBT)

CBT is a form of psychological therapy that focuses on modifying dysfunctional cognitions (thoughts) and examining the link to the feelings these thoughts cause.

There is some evidence that CBT can be useful in the early period of dementia to assist a person with making changes to their thinking and how they are approaching the condition. As the dementia worsens the ability to remember and retain these changes diminishes.

Other forms of talk therapy and reminiscence may prove helpful for the person with dementia to engage in life review. See *Psychological therapies*.

Cognitive distortions

This is a term that has become popularized by cognitive behavioural therapy. These are simply patterns of thinking that don't work but seem as if they do. It is distorted thinking. See *All-or-nothing thinking*, *Catastrophizing*.

Cognitive rehabilitation (CR)

CR is included in the World Health Organization's *Package of Interventions for Rehabilitation* (2023).

The idea that people with dementia could benefit from rehabilitation efforts has taken root in the past two decades. CR is a form of therapy that relies on the neuroplasticity of the brain. If you provide the brain with stimulation that is targeted to specific abilities, repeated in a specific manner, you can improve function in skills that require rebuilding. This approach is used for people with traumatic brain injury and for people with dementia.

The goal is to restore skills and to build skills that assist in compensation for other skills that may have decreased. It is a well-researched approach and should be considered among the range of ways you support the person you care for.

Cognitive stimulation therapy (CST)

There is a growing evidence-base for the effectiveness of this form of dementia therapy for people with mild to moderate dementia.

CST was developed in the UK and uses stimulation to promote well-being and slow the decline in mental functions using our current understanding of neuroplasticity. Mental stimulation and repetition promote brain growth and change. CST is usually delivered in a group setting where the stimulation of social interaction provides opportunity for discussion, sharing of ideas and perspectives, memories and plans.

Activities may include word games, reminiscence, discussion of current events, hobbies such as painting or drawing, and singing, all tailored to the preferences and interests of participants.

These activities are provided for a group of participants over several weeks and may include ongoing maintenance groups after a course of sessions over several months.

Collaboration

This is one of the four relationship styles on the relationship compass (Part I). This is a vital stance to take when working with anyone with dementia, regardless of the progress of the condition. Collaboration is about working together. This is more productive in the long run than doing all the work yourself and presenting completed tasks that you have done for the person.

Collaboration enables a person with dementia to participate, to contribute and so use their intact skills and activate memories, to practise something, and to enjoy a sense of achievement.

Tom Kitwood describes collaboration as 'a deliberate abstinence from the use of power, and hence from all forms of imposition and coercion' (Kitwood, 2019, p.144). It requires a willingness to work alongside as an equal contributor, recognizing that the person with dementia has something to contribute and can do so given sufficient space.

Collaboration builds relationships of trust and mutual regard. These are an integral component of person-centred caring. The alternative is to do for the person and risk them losing their remaining skills through lack of use. The house may be clean and the person well-dressed but do they trust you and are they happy? Are they compliant and passive because they know that to protest is futile?

Comfort

This emotional and physical need is discussed in detail in Part I, along with the other fundamental needs.

Communication

Much is written throughout this book about communication. It is vital to the success of your caregiving with a person with dementia. Good communication is science and art. Given that they will have impairments in their ability to communicate their wants and needs, their preferences, it falls to you to take responsibility for the success of the communication between you both. The further they progress in their condition and the more impaired they become, the more you will need to contribute to the success of the communication.

Successful communication in dementia care relies on an ability to read the person. This means noticing their signals for mood and intention in the content of what they say, their tone of voice and pace of speech. Also look for body language in gestures, facial expression, gait and posture.

Listen to the meaning of what they say. It may not make sense at a superficial level, but if you know the person you may be able infer what they want or intend from clues in the words they use. This is where the art of communicating with someone with dementia comes to the fore. Keep trying until you hit the jackpot. You will know you have correctly understood the person when they settle and stop trying to get their message across to you.

Competence, legal

As dementia progresses, there will come a time when the person with dementia you care for is no longer deemed legally competent. This is a legal step and not a reflection on the person's ability to function in daily concerns at home or socially. This is often a difficult step for the person with dementia and for you. It is difficult emotionally as it can signal a shift in relationship and a shift in self-perception for the person with dementia. They may have difficulty accepting this change in their circumstances.

Competency is, however, not a yes or no attribute. It depends on the situation, the task and the support. A person may have a capacity to perform daily personal care tasks, domestic tasks, or hold a conversation with someone who is attuned to their needs. However, they may not have insight into complex financial matters such as the implications of signing a mortgage or business contract.

They may be able to participate in medical decision-making so long as they have the appropriate support and explanation to help them make sense of the situation. They may be legally not competent to do the above complex tasks but competent to go shopping with you and complete purchases. They may be competent to do this only if you are present, scaffolding the steps in the process so they can be successful. It depends on the situation, the task and the support.

Compliments, praise

We flourish with positive feedback. It feeds our soul. Some people are dependent on it and crave it, while others live quite nicely without it. Whatever the preferences of the person you care for, your positive feedback will have a positive effect on the person. It can lift their mood, help them engage more, and encourage them to attempt tasks they might not otherwise have the confidence to try. Your gratitude can also be affirming as it recognizes them and sends a message that you value what they have done.

Affirm the behaviour you want more of and don't give attention to the behaviour you want less of.

Examples of positive feedback or praise or compliments include: You look lovely in that dress/suit. That's great. Well done. Thanks for helping. Your hair looks terrific. You look handsome.

Confabulation

See *Telling lies*

Consent

Consent is an important topic in all areas of society and is crucial to consider when caring for someone with dementia. Consent is too often assumed in dementia care. Daily activities such as bathing, eating, dressing, all involve consent or agreement to participate. However, just because a person with dementia goes along with you does not mean they have given consent. It may be that they are passively or fearfully cooperating. We know enough about how people react to traumatic assault to recognize that passive cooperation can be an indicator of the freezing fear response. It is not necessarily consent.

The question to ask yourself is: Am I seeing signs/behaviours that indicate engagement with me and active agreement to continue participating? If there is active agreement in a process such as dressing or showering, you will see eye contact, posture or leaning in to you or turning toward you, smiling, a tone of voice indicating calmness and interest, readiness for the next step.

If these signals are not present you may need to ask if they are okay to start or continue. If this is not possible for the person with dementia due to difficulty understanding speech, consider changing the activity and then coming back to it, and watch for signals of active agreement to participate.

Consequences

This topic has been explored extensively in Part I of this book as part of the *ABC model of behaviour management*.

Continence

See also *Bedwetting*

Continence can become an issue in dementia as brain diseases impair self-awareness and self-monitoring. Muscle control may also become impaired.

There are various behavioural management approaches that may be helpful. First is scheduled toileting. This consists of a regular approach by a caregiver to prompt the person to consider using the toilet. It is the regularity of the prompt and subsequent toileting that is important in effectively training the bladder/bowel to expect regular emptying/evacuation. The muscle experience provides feedback to the brain and it adjusts initiation of the urge.

How the response is handled is important because the person with dementia may be initially resistant, but on a second approach or an oblique approach a few minutes later, you may be successful.

Another way is to make it attractive. With my three-year-old granddaughter, my follow-up to my initial prompt and her denial that she needs to go is to sometimes say to her, 'I bet I can get there before you can!' This usually results in her abandoning what she is doing to sprint to the toilet and beat grandpa. Undressing and sitting on the toilet is a natural next step once she is there.

However, this is not advisable for older adults with compromised mobility. I hope you take the idea that you can make going to the toilet attractive. Use honey rather than vinegar, as the old saying goes. You can make it an opportunity to read to them while they sit. 'Would you like to hear the next chapter while you are on the toilet?' This might sound bizarre but you will be surprised how well it works. You leave the door open, or perhaps ajar if privacy is an issue, and you sit outside the toilet/bathroom and read, or sing, or recite poetry. Whatever works! Have you ever played chess with someone sitting on a toilet?

Nocturnal *incontinence* is a real problem for many couples whose shared bed may become impossible to maintain once the person with dementia begins to lose continence. This may be the cause of sleeping in separate beds and for much grief about the loss of this shared part of your lives. It may be a treasured place of closeness and this can be a significant loss and a confirmation of the transition that can occur from wife/husband to caregiver.

Alternatively, it may be a relief to put an end to a feature of your lives together that you have never enjoyed. In this case nocturnal incontinence can be a blessing in disguise. It still needs some response so that the person with dementia is able to continue to sleep without discomfort. There are many types of continence aids on the market and this should be explored among your supports to find what meets your needs. You will likely need to protect the mattress and have a sufficient supply of sheets to enable you to meet the need for fresh linen.

Skin integrity can be compromised if a person is left in a urine-filled continence aid for long. Ensure you obtain advice from a continence specialist about the best procedure, lotions, and so on, so that the person you care for is comfortable and their skin condition is maintained. In the past few years many new products have come on to the market, improving continence care.

Faecal incontinence can be a significant hygiene problem but more of a social problem. You may become adept at taking with you a change of clothing or at least underwear when you go out if faecal incontinence is likely.

It is better to try to manage the incontinence so that it doesn't occur – if possible. The areas you can have some effect on include diet and regularity. If you live with the person with dementia you can have an influence over what the person eats. The diet should have a balance that ensures firm stools. Loose bowel motions make it difficult for the person with dementia to 'read' the signals from their body that they need to go to the toilet. If they have firm stools, their brains are more likely to receive strong signals that a bowel action is needed. This can lead to appropriate well-learned toileting behaviour.

Cleaning up after a bowel accident can be a difficult task if you have not been used to doing it since your children were small. It can also be accompanied by a sense of disgust and perhaps anger that the person with dementia has done this. Blaming can come quickly if you are not careful to manage your feelings. Blame is harmful to the person with dementia, who may feel a sense of shame already at having an accident. It is the dementia that is responsible for this problem, not the person with dementia.

It can happen that the person tries to clean themselves up after a faecal accident and makes it worse by spreading faeces over themselves, walls and other objects they touch. This requires a level head and patience from you. Offer them one of the many types of disposable wipes so they can clean their hands and then give them a drink or something else to hold while you go about changing their clothes and cleaning them up further. All the while keep up a stream of chat about a topic that engages them without too much effort. This is important to ensure that they are in touch with your mood through your tone of voice – after an event like this they can tend to feel shame and be angry with themselves and perhaps project that anger on to you being angry with them. Keep talking to them in a calm, neutral way and gradually they will calm and be ready to move to the next thing in their day.

See *Incontinence, Bedwetting, Soiling.*

Conversation

This is an important activity that stimulates the person with dementia to think, find words, participate in turn-taking and exercise their memory. Try to find ways to activate conversation so that the person with dementia is stimulated to remember, think, problem-solve and contribute. Ask questions, get them thinking. Ask for their thoughts. Let them know that what they have to offer is valued and important. Conversation is stimulating for the brain and provides opportunities for connection and emotional closeness.

Cooperation

Cooperation is vital for success in dementia caring. This requires ingenuity, patience and acceptance from you as caregiver. But mostly it requires a willingness to work together with the person with dementia.

It also applies to local supports, cooperating with other people locally who are carers for someone with dementia. Get together to share ideas and problems so you can learn from their efforts and they from yours. This also helps to overcome the social isolation that can come with caregiving. Online groups are more important than ever for support and a sense of shared endeavour. You may not have been a 'joiner' but now is the time to join groups to support each other.

Coordination problems

Eventually mobility will be affected by the progress of dementia. When the brain does not reliably send signals to move or not move to the muscles, you will see coordination or movement difficulties. This can affect gait and result in falling over or tripping. It can also show in the fine motor control required to eat, clean teeth, write, paint, draw, grip and grasp objects, and wash and dry oneself. When combined with balance, this problem of coordination can produce injuries or breakages. It is wise to obtain an assessment with a physiotherapist and/or occupational therapist as soon as possible so the problems can be identified accurately and early, and strategies to assist can be designed.

Creativity

Having dementia can be a freeing experience in which creativity is released and can be expressed perhaps for the first time in a person's life. If you as carer are in tune with this need you can support the person's creative effort by providing the time, physical space and the means for them to express this creativity. In other words, you can scaffold the experience so they are successful. You don't have to join it but sometimes doing that can provide just the stimulus a person needs in order to engage in a new task. Once they see you having a go they can feel emboldened to have a go themselves. They may also copy your actions initially (mirroring) and then continue without needing the scaffolding of your actions to remain engaged.

Cynicism

Cynicism in caregivers occurs as a defence against the feelings that arise when caring closely for someone with dementia. It may include dismissing loving feelings or tears. Or it may be anger about the cost of caregiving to one's own life or about the change in the relationship with the person you love. It may be sadness in response to seeing a person you love experience such changes as occur in dementia. Sadness is usually a response to loss and it signals how much what is lost means to you. Cynicism keeps these feelings buried or at the least unacknowledged. If this happens, it may not be long before you become depressed, with explosive moments followed by periods of self-blame.

If you find yourself becoming cynical you may need to talk to a support person who can help you find a way to acknowledge the feelings that come with caregiving.

Dad

Father figures can be sources of great comfort and reassurance. They can be associated with feeling confident to have a go at tasks. As a carer, you can utilize your knowledge of the person's father to judge if this is the case for them and how it could be used to help them feel better about themselves and attempt various tasks.

If you are a male carer with a person with dementia, you may be associated with their father. So depending on what their father was like you may find yourself the subject of projections onto you. These projections can be of a past, long-deceased but emotionally significant parent. You may be mistaken for the parent figure, spoken to and treated as if you are the parent figure. If you are a male spouse/carer, you may activate associations with the father that are a mix of pleasant and unpleasant connections with past and very early life experience.

If it is physically safe to do so and the person is not distressed by their sense of you as their parent, maintain dialogue in a comforting or positive manner. Avoid contradicting or correcting the person. This will only result in a conflict in which there can be only one winner – you. You may also risk that the person with dementia may disengage and withdraw, feeling as though they have made a mistake – got it wrong again.

Dance

Dance can be a good way to engage the person with dementia in an activity that takes them out of their thinking and into bodily movement. You may be surprised how the rhythm of dance can remain intact and be stimulated simply by playing music. Even though speech and language skills may have become impaired, it is possible that well-learned dances from younger years may be accessible and provide opportunities for enjoyment and relaxation. It is possible that dance may offer a circuit breaker if tension is high between you both.

If the person you care for is open to it, it may be useful to attend a freestyle dancing group in which the person with dementia can participate with free movement. This can be done on their own without a partner so it may give them freedom to express mood and feelings in a physical way that bypasses language problems.

Death

Depending on the insight and language abilities of the person you care for, death may be a topic of conversation. If this comes up, be open and frank about it. Dementia is a life-shortening condition.

The idea of their own death may cause them concern, in which case reassure them that you will be there with them till the end and that you will take care of them. If it is your death they are concerned about, you may need to ask them what they would like to have happen if you were to die before them. Ideally you have already had this conversation, but plans can change and need to be adaptable to different circumstances.

You may find that it upsets them too much to hear of family or friends who die, in which case try to judge the person's capacity to handle the information, for instance, that a loved one has died and adjust what you say to what you believe they can manage without becoming overwhelmed. You may then use whatever ways you usually use to avoid going near an emotionally difficult topic.

This is relevant to the issue of telling the truth to people with dementia. I tend to err on the side of truth telling rather than deceiving by omission. However, it is a matter for judgement in your individual circumstances. People with dementia can adjust to unpleasant information and despite forgetfulness can, with repetition, retain traces of the information, particularly if it is emotionally important to them.

So my usual approach is to tell the person the unpleasant news, stick around for the emotional fallout and provide support and gentle repetition if necessary as they come to grips with it, and be ready to help them go on with their day. Perhaps stimulate memories of the person who has died with conversation or photographs.

Don't be afraid of emotional upset. Emotions come and go. What remains is the sense of connection, acceptance and care.

Decision-making

People with dementia should be encouraged and supported to continue decision-making as long as they are able. Making decisions is a vital part of functioning as a human being. We teach it to small children and we support and shape their capacity to make decisions that are kind and thoughtful, safe and respectful.

Making decisions supports confidence and a sense of control over one's world. Decisions enable a sense of agency that maintains function as an equal, a participant in the social milieu.

For as long as the person with dementia has language skills that enable them to comprehend your speech, you will be able to ask them directly what they prefer and keep them engaged in decision-making. When the time comes and language is less reliable, you may need to rely on non-verbal cues to elicit preferences and engage the other person in making choices.

Simplify the choices offered to what they can be successful with. For instance, an open question ('What would you like for lunch?') is the most cognitively complex one to answer as it requires an ability to think of a range of possibilities and choose from among them. A closed question is less cognitively complex ('Would you like a sandwich for lunch?') and requires only a choice between yes and no.

Decision-making invites the person with dementia to participate in normal human activity and this supports a sense of self, and confidence in oneself, and provides opportunities for enjoyment that might not be otherwise possible. Remember that they are living their lives, not yours.

Physical safety is about the only reason we as caregivers need to step in and take over a situation. And even then, it requires explanation and defusing if your controlling action causes resentment.

Defences

Defences or defence mechanisms are unconscious patterns of emotion and behaviour that protect you from feeling anxiety or keep aspects of yourself from awareness that would be upsetting to acknowledge. A selection of defences commonly seen in dementia care are examined under the individual defence.

See *Denial*, *Repression* and *Regression*.

Defensiveness

This is the sign that a psychological or emotional defence has been stimulated and the person does not want to acknowledge or engage with the situation – the person experiences self-anger at realizing they have made a mistake.

Delusions

Delusions are fixed, false ideas. They occur commonly in the course of dementia, sometimes accompanied by sensory *hallucinations*. This happens as the person's brain attempts to make sense of the world with diminishing mental resources.

Your behaviour may become incorporated into a delusion. You may be perceived as a thief who takes their possessions and puts them where they cannot find them. Or as a jailer who restricts them from leaving the house.

Types of delusions can include:

- being paranoid (suspicious, doubtful of others)
- persecution (you make my life difficult, you hurt me)
- control (a force makes me do things)
- reference (the numbers on a licence plate mean the end of the world is coming)
- being grandiose (I have a special mission in life).

If the person with dementia has a delusion, do not try to argue against it to prove how it is false. This will only reinforce the belief and create distress for them.

Empathize with their feeling-state rather than debate the truth of their belief. Being understood and calmed will be more help to them. For instance, if they feel agitated by the belief you may say, 'I am sorry this has upset you so much', or, 'I am sorry you are so worried.' You position yourself as a trusted companion at a time when they may be suspicious and wary.

Medication may be a solution to help minimize the distress but it should always be used with specialist medical advice and reviewed regularly.

Delirium

Delirium is not dementia. Delirium is a short-term change in consciousness and general brain function that is caused by infections, alcohol, imbalances in electrolytes, dehydration, medication and kidney failure, to name a few. It is reversible, dementia is not.

The most common cause of delirium is urinary tract infection. This can cause not only physical pain but confusion, agitation, restlessness and behavioural and mood disturbance. Typically, symptoms fluctuate. It has a rapid onset and generally a long tail of symptoms, even after the infection has been treated. Treatment is antibiotics. Avoid the cause by monitoring for good personal hygiene and ensuring that the person with dementia cleans themselves adequately after using the toilet and washes their hands.

Other sources of delirium are infections of chest, ears and gums. Good oral hygiene (see *Teeth*) and regular check-ups at the dentist can be important to avoid gum infections. If you notice a relatively quick change in level of confusion, agitation, restlessness, or an increase in hallucinations, seek medical assessment to rule out delirium or obtain treatment. The earlier you obtain medical treatment for the cause, the better will be the recovery. Maintain fluid intake and nourishment too.

As a caregiver you can help by creating a calm, quiet and well-lit physical environment. Be patient with symptoms of confusion or agitation. It is medical, not personal. Keep instructions simple.

Dementia

Dementia is a progressive, irreversible condition caused by a range of diseases of the brain. It is characterized by decline in all brain functions. These include thinking, memory, problem-solving, personality and behaviour. The most common cause of dementia is *Alzheimer's disease*.

Dementia is the leading cause of disease burden in those over the age of 65 years. The number of Australians with dementia is predicted to almost double by 2058 (Australian Institute of Health and Welfare, 2024). Most other western countries also predict a doubling in the diagnoses of dementia.

While the commonest cause of dementia is *Alzheimer's disease*, vascular disease, Parkinson's disease, Lewy body disease, fronto-temporal disease and chronic alcohol or other drug abuse also contribute to its prevalence. Other less common forms of dementia can be caused by conditions including: Huntington's disease, progressive supranuclear palsy, Creutzfeldt–Jakob disease and HIV-associated neurocognitive disorder. If you require more detailed information about these conditions there is a wealth of information readily available on the internet.

Dementia is characterized by:

- memory loss

- impairments in language expression and comprehension, object recognition, task performance

- personality change

- executive dysfunction such as disinhibition, and problems with organization, planning, sequencing, abstract thought and problem-solving.

These symptoms cause significant social and behavioural changes. The changes reduce capacity to function independently and confidently. In the middle-to-later phases of the condition, symptoms frequently result in admission to residential care homes. Consequently, people with dementia can experience separation from family and past life, which can make relocation all the harder.

See also *Younger onset dementia*.

Denial

Denial is one of the major psychological defences used by people with dementia to defend against unwanted or unacceptable information about themselves in an effort to maintain their self-esteem or self-image. If making errors has been unacceptable to them throughout their lives this may continue through the period that they have dementia. This defensiveness may involve them putting the blame on to you. This involves a denial and displacement of responsibility on to you. It involves simply refusing to acknowledge the existence of the unacceptable information. *You* must have forgotten to do it (whatever it was). *You* put the knives in the wrong drawer, the milk in the pantry, the keys in the fridge. *You* stole the money from my wallet.

If someone is denying responsibility for their mistakes, confronting them head-on will only make the denial stronger. Do not argue whether this is true or not. Arguing only reinforces the person's belief in the statement and they will 'dig their heels in'. Better to come at it from another angle: 'Okay, well let's look for your purse. Maybe it was dropped on the way out.' Or if they want to report it to the police, you can offer to accompany them to the police station to make a report. More often than not the person will not want to follow through on this and you may be able to conduct a search of the house while they sleep and then place the recovered item where they can find it on waking.

Dentist

See *Teeth*

Depression

Depression is more common among people who have dementia than among the general population, with rates of up to 60 per cent. There is some evidence for late onset depression being an early sign of dementia and a risk factor for it. Symptoms include loss of interest in previously enjoyed activities, lack of motivation, low mood, changes in appetite and sleep, and being preoccupied with past wrongs and guilt.

Treatment in older adults is most often medication (see *Antidepressant medication*).

However, if people with dementia have language skills and memory still available, they may benefit from psychotherapy or talk therapy. Modified forms of talk therapy for older adults with dementia (shorter sessions, life review) can be an effective form of help.

Regular exercise is one of the most effective treatments for depression. Other approaches may include sticking to routines, engaging in previously enjoyed activities and roles. It is the loss of these that often contributes to depression in dementia as the person loses confidence and opportunity once dementia is diagnosed. As a carer, try to maintain function and role as much as possible for as long as possible.

Dignity

Dignity is a vital quality of one's subjective sense of self. One's dignity is often sadly diminished in dementia by dependence on others for assistance with previously achievable tasks.

In the person-centred approach to dementia care it is an indicator of one's personhood to be held intact and affirmed or enhanced. Dignity can be affirmed and supported by addressing the person with the title or name they prefer, appropriate to your relationship to them. It may be simply your tone of respect in your speech to them that says, 'I recognize your value.' It can be affirmed as a caregiver by utilizing information you know about the person to indicate to them that you value some quality or aspect of their experience.

For instance, you may call them Mrs or Mr. You may refer to their wartime experience, but this can be difficult if they do not want it referred to by strangers. It comes down to your relationship with them. If you are the spouse of a person with dementia you may know that wartime remembrance can be a cause of bad dreams and moodiness, or it may be a time to go through photo albums to reminisce about former comrades in arms.

Disempowerment

When you take over or do tasks for the person with dementia that they could do themselves or with some assistance, you disempower them. You take their power away. You also inadvertently speed up the process of dementia by preventing them from using the skills and knowledge they have. Remaining skills require daily use to remain available. If you take over for convenience or out of habit, you disempower and rob the person of their skills and knowledge. If you do this often enough or see others do it, you may notice that a person with dementia either loses the motivation to even try or becomes angry and upset at being denied the chance to do what they can.

See *Empowerment*.

Disparagement

Criticism can be destructive of selfhood. You know yourself that when you have been criticized in your life it sticks. It has a disproportionate negative effect on self-esteem. Avoid all disparaging comments or criticism toward a person with dementia. The experience of making mistakes and forgetting is frequent for them and feeling bad about themselves is just around the corner most of the time. If you can't be affirming or neutral it may be best to stay silent. If you are angry or frustrated you may need to take time out.

Disruption

Interruptions can occur many times in your day. You adjust and roll with it. However, for a person with dementia, the effect of a disruption can be to stop them doing something enjoyable and not be able to re-engage with it. Disruptions occur when your agenda becomes more important than the focus on the person with dementia. Medication has to be taken, preparation for a shopping trip interrupts mealtime, or toilet stops singing.

Be wary of disrupting whatever the person with dementia is engaged in just because it is your agenda for how the day should go. Stop yourself and ask, 'Do I need to interrupt/disrupt the person or can it wait?' If it can wait, bide your time and do it in the break or natural pause between activities.

What you want to do is no more important than what the person with dementia wants to do.

Distraction

Distraction is a useful way of directing the attention of a person with dementia away from a negative focus to a more positive experience or focus. If they are becoming fixed on the desire to go for a walk and it is pouring with rain, it may be useful to use distraction.

See 'Distraction/Redirection' (in 'Behavioural approaches to use', Part I) for a full discussion of the use of distraction.

Distress behaviour

Many names have been used over the years for the behaviour of a person with dementia. These include problem behaviour, disruptive behaviour, challenging behaviour, difficult behaviour and, of course, behavioural and psychological symptoms of dementia (BPSD). A recent adaptation is responsive behaviour, which indicates that the person with dementia may be responding to something rather than just being difficult, challenging or disruptive.

The most recent and perhaps most humane term is *distress behaviour*. This indicates that to behave in an aggressive, repetitive, anxious or upset way the person must be in a state of distress. If a person feels happy and content, they are not likely to be aggressive, repetitive, anxious or upset. Distress behaviour points you in the direction of analysis and problem-solving when considering the issue that is causing the distress.

It has been suggested elsewhere in this book that the distress can be attributed to events in relationships that evoke a person's attachment predisposition. This can be a useful place to begin if you are a caregiver and trying to work out why a person is behaving in a particular way. Could their aggression be an indicator of attachment distress; do they feel abandoned or smothered, anxious or needing reassurance? If so, attention to their attachment preferences/needs will provide a way forward in responding to their needs. See *Attachment*.

Disturbed behaviour

See *Problem behaviour*, *Challenging behaviour* and *Distress behaviour*

Domestic tasks

Everyday tasks around the home are important for a person with dementia to be able to continue to do as they are usually so well learned that they are automatic or over-learned. They require little or no conscious attention to complete successfully. Such tasks include washing clothes, washing dishes, drying dishes, setting the table, clearing the table of plates, sweeping the floor, vacuuming, opening/closing the blinds/curtains, taking out the rubbish/bins.

By using skills, you maintain existing brain pathways and reinforce them with repetition. This works against the deteriorating effects of the disease causing the dementia and slows it down. It also helps the person feel competent and more likely to want to remain a participant and useful.

The person you care for may require support to be successful. Keep a watchful eye on the steps for which they need your assistance. Provide only enough help for them to resume independent function. Then back off and be there to offer affirmation at the end. Bear in mind that some people need a lot of praise and some don't want any. Adapt your affirmation to what *they* need, not what you feel like offering.

Double entendre

A double entendre is a word or phrase that has a double meaning, with one meaning usually indecent or risqué. To understand a double entendre, you need to have an ability to see both meanings at once. For a person with dementia this is frequently difficult and can cause misunderstandings and frustration for them.

The reason these are difficult is that the ability to process language, particularly understanding the meaning of words, becomes impaired. The person with dementia may be more inclined to interpret what you say literally as this is easier and more obvious than an oblique or abstract reference.

My suggestion is to avoid these word plays all together. Keep language as straightforward as possible.

Dressing

Getting dressed is something you have done all your life since about the age of two years. It has become so automatic that you need only think consciously about which shirt among several to put on rather than how to do it and what order to do it in. Or even what to do with a piece of clothing in front of you.

Getting dressed is an important task that needs to be done successfully for social acceptance, self-image, modesty and comfort. In dementia, a person may have impairments that affect their ability to initiate or complete the task of dressing.

You can help by preparing clothing in the correct order for them to put on so they can dress with underwear on first. Lay the clothes out on the bed so they can see what is what and take up the underwear first. If the person you care for wants to contribute their choices to dressing you might want to offer simple choices such as: 'Would you like to wear this one or this one [holding up two shirts]?' An even simpler question is: 'Would you like to wear this one [holding up one shirt]? Avoid open choices as these are usually too perplexing. However, if the person can cope with an open question ('What would you like to wear today?') and can successfully exercise choice, by all means use an open question.

It is important to dress for the weather. The person with

dementia may not have an awareness of the weather as they dress unless you introduce it to them. 'It's a warm day today so perhaps a shirt and shorts may be good. See what you think.'

Particular occasions require certain dress and it is important that the person with dementia does not stand out to attract ridicule or disparagement because of their dress choice. Social inclusion is difficult to maintain for people with dementia, without attracting negative commentary that can be avoided.

That said, if all your efforts to encourage the person to dress for the occasion are fruitless and they stubbornly refuse to wear the suit jacket and tie and prefer a T-shirt and jeans, then go with what is possible. There is no point causing the person to feel angry with you for the sake of a suit. So, the bottom line is: try to achieve your goal but not at the cost of their well-being.

If the person has previously dressed in an idiosyncratic manner then their clothing choices may not be all that different from their pre-dementia choices.

Driving

This is a fraught topic. However, some simple guidelines may help. The safety of the community is paramount. Therefore, if the person with dementia is not able to drive safely, their licence should be cancelled. Their safety can be determined by a qualified occupational therapist (or similar in your country). Such an assessment can be arranged through their general practitioner (GP). How you go about this process matters a great deal.

If as a caregiver you have concerns about their driving safety, it is responsible to begin a conversation with them about that. Usually this will be met with some resistance to the idea that they may not be able to drive safely. Go gently but keep your goal clear – the safety of the community.

Driving may have meaning for the person with dementia, such as a way to maintain independence, and the loss of driving may signal the beginning of the end of an independent life for them. Giving up driving may also signal a new balance in their relationship with you if you are to take up the driving now. They become the passenger, perhaps for the first time in your relationship. See if you can engage in a conversation about what driving means to

LIVING WITH A PERSON WITH DEMENTIA

them. This will help them, and you, to be clear about why they are resisting the idea of not driving.

If necessary, go to or write to the GP so that they can introduce the idea of a driving assessment to the person you care for. This way you can avoid being 'the bad guy'.

Remain as sympathetic as you can about the cost of giving up driving but also stay steadfast about safety of the community. Some things are not negotiable and at some depth they will see the point of your concern. Plan ahead so that they have enough time to come to grips with it and are not bulldozed into it.

Dying

See *Palliative care*

Eating

Food is a central part of life for us all. For people living with dementia, mealtime is a welcome activity that is engaging and enjoyable and helps to punctuate the day. It's a time to stop together, communicate and look at each other. It's so much more than food.

As a home carer, you can take up the opportunity that mealtimes present, to make them key moments of the day. Breakfast is a transition from sleep to awake, a gentle, quiet time for planning the day ahead or reiterating what the day holds so the person with dementia is oriented to what is happening next.

Small nutrition and hydration breaks for juice and a snack can then punctuate an activity and provide moments of rest. Then lunch is an opportunity to refuel and announce what is happening next or simply revisit the morning to enjoy it some more.

The evening meal signals the end of the day and a restful transition from activity to quiet wind-down.

You may need to provide physical assistance with meals but only enough to ensure that the person is ingesting their food. If the person you care for is physically capable of eating independently, they may require only a verbal prompt to keep eating: 'How is the soup?' Alternatively, they may require food to be cut up or to be presented on a fork or spoon. If you are presenting food to be eaten, do it at a pace and in a manner that preserves the person's dignity – wait until they swallow the previous mouthful before presenting the next. Don't hold the loaded spoon outside their mouth like a helicopter waiting to dash in. Ensure that the amount of food is small enough that there is no need to repeatedly wipe the excess off their face. Do it with dignity and respect.

Have minimal noise and other stimuli in the eating area so that they can concentrate on the task at hand. Music is fine to relax with but can be a distraction and overwhelming if the person with dementia has reduced concentration or attention resources.

When assisting the person to eat, sit so that they can see you and you can easily see them swallow.

If you eat with them, they are more likely to mirror your behaviour and initiate eating themselves (see *Mirroring*). Mirroring like this can be a real help in starting the person off, particularly if they have frontal lobe impairment that diminishes motivation to commence an activity (see *Adynamia*). They may effectively borrow your motivation and initiative to commence eating.

If the person is unable to sit to eat due to agitation and restlessness, you may need to develop a finger-food selection so they can maintain nourishment without the stress of being restricted to a chair to eat (see *Finger-food*).

Emotions

Emotions are vital human experiences that enable you to experience the world and react to it. Depending on who you ask, they include anger, sadness, joy, disgust, fear and love. Anger helps you to know what is a threat and react to it in an active way. Sadness lets you know when you have lost someone you love or something important so you can grieve it. Joy helps you to celebrate your pleasure and the world around you. Disgust helps you to know what food to avoid and what situations you find toxic. Fear helps you to move away from danger. Love helps you to move towards others who you find attractive and want to be involved with and to whom you wish to be committed. All emotions serve a purpose that enhances your life.

If you search 'emotions' on the internet you will find various lists and ways of explaining what emotions are and how they differ from feelings. The above lists the basic emotions that seem to appear in most lists. In the simplest terms, emotions are sensations in the body that register with the brain. Anger is heat in the chest that rises from the gut, activating the large muscles, blood pressure, pulse rate and breathing, in readiness for action. The brain registers this process and reinforces it as it interprets the visual and auditory signals that confirm there is a threat to respond to.

Feelings, on the other hand, are generated by our thoughts and use emotional information but are often not accurate. For example, we learn to regard anger and sadness as negative emotions. So, we tell ourselves to avoid them. We learn this early in our families. In common speech, we use these two terms interchangeably. People with dementia will use the words emotion and feelings as we all do, which is not very accurately. Which term you use is largely unimportant in everyday use, as long as you understand that emotions are the physical experience that we often are unaware of and feelings are the interpretation of this experience based on our personal background and life experiences.

When dementia occurs, feelings can gradually become less controlled by the learned thinking and social habits that usually help us to manage our behaviour in society. This can result in emotional storms on the one hand and also a flattening of the expression of emotion on the other. This can be very confusing as a caregiver, as the expression of feelings is an important part of personality style. It can feel as though the person with dementia is no longer the same.

It is important to say here that emotions are not behaviour. We must make a distinction between emotions and the behaviour that can follow the activation of emotion. This is best illustrated with anger and sadness.

Anger is the emotion. It is internal and invisible to an observer. Aggression and violence are behaviours that are visible and audible to an observer. It is neither good nor bad. It is not a moral experience. Anger is a physical experience that is a reaction to events around us or to our thoughts and memories. Aggression and violence are what we decide to do or say as a result of the emotional experience. We may not be conscious of deciding, as it is very quick, but it is there. Whatever we decide to do, the basis of feeling angry can be good for us and others around us, or not.

It is the emotional experience that gives rise to crying behaviour, tears, running nose, holding our face, withdrawal from others. What we decide to do on the basis of feeling sad can be good for us, or not.

It is also useful to add here that the experience of emotion can make us anxious, depending on our personal background. The signs of anxiety are frequently misinterpreted as anger. Tight chest, palpitations, raised heart rate and dry mouth are all signs of anxiety. All of these are often misreported as indications of anger.

You may have noticed that anxiety was not listed among emotions in the list above. This is because it is frequently a defensive reaction to emotion, in that we become anxious when we have anger or sadness, and so on. There is no external threat to be anxious about. The danger is perceived as coming from within. The defensive response is to push it down, deny it, distract ourselves from it, or detach and act as if it isn't there.

Alternatively, our response may be to explode and discharge it towards others in rage or tears. This emotional discharge decreases inner tension about the presence of the emotion. We feel calmer and often regret the discharge and can feel shame and embarrassment.

For people with dementia, this latter reaction is most common as they can become confused and overwhelmed by the rise of emotions within themselves and discharge the emotion to relieve the rising tension that comes with it.

As a caregiver, your role can be to keep the person safe, to avoid condemning them with negative responses, and reassure them. It may also be to protect them from negative social feedback that can come in the form of criticism from others if they have exploded verbally.

Empathy

This is the ability to feel and understand what another person is feeling. It is the basis for us as humans being able to have compassion for one another, for kindness and caregiving. Empathy is an essential ability that helps you to identify the feelings of another person. It then enables you to adjust your caregiving to meet the needs of the other person. Some of us are very empathic and others less so. Wherever you find yourself on the spectrum of empathy, you can improve your skill at it by watching for facial expression and tone of voice changes that signal changes in feelings. This can be your clue to the emotional experience of the other person.

See also *Mirroring*.

Empowerment

Empowerment is one of the positive care actions identified by Tom Kitwood (1997) as promoting and sustaining well-being. To empower another person requires *empathy* and the ability to manage your own desire to control the outcome in a caregiving situation. To empower means to allow or support the other person to act with power, influence and agency. It requires you to step back and scaffold the other person's effort rather than do it yourself.

Examples of empowerment include: handing the person a spoon to eat with if they are having difficulty with a fork; waiting a little longer than you are tempted to, so the person can find a way to put their trousers on themselves; arranging the clothing on the bed in the order in which they have to put it on.

This is an essential skill in dementia caregiving as it supports the function of the person for as long as possible. If the person has to use all their abilities to function as much as possible, their brains will have to find a way to do the task. Repeated challenge to find a way is what enables a person to remember, to understand and to use skills and knowledge. Empowerment is vital for well-being.

End of life

See *Palliative care*

Enjoyment

Moments of enjoyment are an important part of the mix of daily life. Caring for a person with dementia can become focused on the practical tasks necessary to enable the person to get through the day. However, if you can also create or take moments to enjoy life together, you will find less burden and some lightness in the daily routines.

These can be moments of singing a song together in the shower, or telling a story of past holidays or funny moments from the past with your children. These stimulate memory and pleasure.

Ethics

There are many ethical issues raised by having dementia and providing care to a person living with dementia. Some of these issues include: how to protect the person with dementia without disempowering them; how to enable the person without creating risks to physical safety; how to facilitate freedom of movement safely; monitoring the person's movements without being 'big brother' and taking away their freedom; deciding whether to tell the truth or not when it may create distress for a person with dementia; how to speak to a person with dementia without infantilizing them.

A book I have found particularly helpful is *The Moral Challenge of Alzheimer Disease: Ethical Issues from Diagnosis to Dying* by Stephen G. Post (2000). It is easy to read and you can dip in and out of it as you need. The growth in technology, particularly in wearables, is not examined in depth but it remains the best exploration of ethical issues related to dementia care. Post speaks of 'the deeply forgetful' when referring to people with dementia. It is a respectful and compassionate way to refer to people whose lives have been turned upside down by this condition.

Wearables are personal electronic devices (watches, personal alarms, earbuds and tracking devices) that allow you or others to monitor a person's performance or whereabouts. Applied to people living with dementia, their use raises issues of personal freedom/autonomy and privacy. There is not enough space to explore this issue here. Suffice to say that it remains unresolved as technology develops quickly. We have not yet developed ethical guidelines for use of such devices in the community let alone among people living with dementia. Until such time as society develops guidelines for use in the wider community, use among people with dementia will remain contentious.

Excess disability

This is a notion that describes the disability a person with dementia may experience due to the way they are spoken to and treated by others, which adds to the disability that can be attributed to the condition.

For example, a person with dementia may become uncertain and unable to find words if they are overwhelmed by a dominating person who speaks to them quickly and demands an answer to a complex question, or gives them lots of information quickly. The person with dementia may seem more disabled than they really are due to the inappropriate communication.

Another example is aggression. A person with dementia may become aggressive if they are dominated or compelled to have a shower or go to the toilet without being invited to or asked. Their reaction is normal to such treatment but may attract negative remarks from others and result in medication to modify their outbursts.

If poor communication occurs constantly throughout a person's time with dementia, their decline in skills may progress more rapidly than it might otherwise.

Sensitive, person-centred communication reduces the likelihood of excess disability.

Executive function

This refers to a group of abilities that enable you to act like an executive. They include: planning, organization, self-regulation, self-awareness, sequencing, handling multiple tasks, focus and attention, memory and problem-solving. These skills are usually associated with frontal lobe function. However, they can also be found in other areas of the brain.

Executive dysfunction is a problem in dementia, particularly in dementias that affect the frontal lobes. Most behavioural difficulties can be tracked back to executive dysfunction in some form. For example, without the ability to regulate what you say, you can find social relationships become unstable as people are upset by your words. You may tend to think it and say it, without the mental filtering that prevents you saying everything you think.

As a caregiver, you may find the person with dementia has a lack of awareness that they have done anything that should upset another person. The lack of social awareness is also part of executive dysfunction. Difficulty sequencing affects multiple-step processes such as dressing or eating. Difficulty planning and organizing affects most personal care and preparation for outings so that carers are required to support and scaffold what were once simple procedures.

Exercise

Physical exercise should not stop with a diagnosis of dementia. It remains a vital part of life and in some ways becomes more important to maintain as the person may not be motivated nor remember to do it themselves. They may become reliant on you to support their physical health by reminding, prompting and then doing the exercises alongside them if necessary.

Caregivers need exercise too! It is an important component of life and you need it no less than the person you are caring for. Ensure that it is part of both your lives.

Facilitation

This is a way to enable a person with dementia to be successful at tasks without you taking over. You make it possible for them to succeed. Much as a Sherpa facilitates the success of a mountain climber, you provide all that is necessary for the other person to succeed. This may take the form of giving just the right amount of instruction, broken down into small steps of a task, or laying out items of clothing in the order the person needs to put them on so that they dress in the correct order.

See *Scaffolding*.

Faith

Faith experience is an important dimension of life for many people. For some, it may involve a religious practice. For others, it's a personal awareness that shapes their sense of self, the world and the purpose of life itself. For some, it may be a combination of both. Faith practice is important to maintain as long as possible for people who have dementia. This may mean you organizing your lives so that the person can attend a church regularly or it may mean arranging for the local pastor, rabbi, imam or priest to visit your house.

Family

Most of us grow up in a family. This small group of people with whom you share a history provides a core of familiarity, a platform from which to engage with the world. For a person with dementia, family may become more and more important as a source of memory prompts that support and stimulates remembering. They know the stories, the meaningful moments, the people who matter to us. Visits by family members are a vital factor for reminiscence, for meaningful engagement with the personal narrative of the person who is unable to connect with their personal story without assistance.

See *Reminiscence, Photographs.*

Fear of strangers

As dementia progresses, a person with dementia may find strangers confusing and anxiety-provoking. It may be that they cannot remember previously familiar people and are confused by their (what feels like) overly familiar approach such as the use of pet names or hugging.

It may also be that the person with dementia wants to stay at home and not mix with people or go to supermarkets or shopping centres. It is important to determine the reason for this reluctance. If it is that they find everyone unfamiliar and confusing, it may be important to shop at times when there are fewer people about and the shops are less busy. It could be that the stimulation of noise and movement is too much to process calmly, in which case quieter shopping times are a solution.

Prepare visitors to your house by telling them to introduce themselves each time they visit, and include a brief statement of how they know the person you care for. This may smooth the initial moments a 'stranger' comes to the house.

Dementia erodes memories for people who were once impor-tant. There may still be traces of memory that can be stimulated with the right story or word, so keep up the prompts. Emotional attachment to familiar people becomes much more important as dementia progresses. If you know a person is going to visit today, it may be helpful to prepare the person with dementia by telling them ahead of time so you lay down a memory trace that they can draw on when the person arrives.

If having people come to the house is too stressful it may be helpful to limit visitors or structure visits so that you can benefit from the stimulation as you need and the person with dementia can find a quiet way to be present in the house without demand or strain.

Fears

Fearfulness can be a difficult experience for people with demen-tia. It is largely due to the unfamiliarity created by memory loss, and by the perceptions of risk and danger. A previously familiar world in which the person has functioned with competence and achievement may now be a source of fear and apprehension.

Support in the form of facilitation, prompts, reminders and gentle reassurance may be sufficient to enable the person to con-tinue functioning in an increasingly unfamiliar and fearsome world. This may take the form of brief explanations and simple prompts to enable them to face one part of a situation at a time. If they trust you, they will be more likely to face the world with some confidence and willingness.

Avoid making a person with dementia do something they are afraid of as it will usually result in them digging their heels in, a breach of trust or, at worst, they might flee the situation.

Feeding

Feeding is something you do for animals in the zoo or livestock. For human beings we assist them to eat.

See *Eating*.

Feelings

Feelings are the cognitive and physical experiences you have when emotions are activated in your body. The thoughts you have when you experience emotions, such as anger, help you evaluate and act in response to whatever stimulated the emotional experience. Anger and sadness are regarded as negative feelings as they can be unpleasant.

However, as noted in the entry *Emotions*, anger and sadness have an evolutionary purpose. Anger helps us to feel strong in response to threat. Sadness helps us to know the importance of what we have lost and to value and remember it.

You may have grown up with negative instructions about feelings. 'You're far too emotional', 'Don't let your emotions get the better of you/get in the way', 'Feelings are for sissies', 'Don't be such a cry baby'.

Gendered beliefs about feelings suggest that to feel your feelings is to be a 'girl' and 'real men don't cry'. Thankfully, some of this gender bias is decreasing but, in some communities, it still holds sway. Among the generations experiencing dementia, gendered instructions about feelings are commonplace. It is sufficient to say that these instructions are false and misleading. Feelings are universal experiences that transcend gender. The social embargoes that tell us that feelings are not okay for some people create anxiety and depression for those who try to restrict their emotional lives.

It is suggested that when people with dementia experience feelings they should be supported to have their experience without you making negative or evaluative comments. Just sit quietly with them and provide comfort or reassurance, and perhaps tissues if necessary.

If a person with dementia becomes aggressive when they feel angry it may be necessary to make them safe by removing sharp or heavy objects or placing something soft in their hands so they cannot do damage to themselves or you. You may need to distract them, use limit setting to contain the aggression, and express understanding of their anger but remind them that aggression is not okay.

Remember also that feelings have a beginning, a middle and

an end. They come and go. The person will settle and return to calm. Just be a companion for them.

See *Emotions, Aggression, Sadness*.

Financial planning

When a person is diagnosed with dementia, a number of actions usually follow with legal, financial and practical consequences.

One of these consequences is that you may have to sort out power-of-attorney documentation so that you can prepare for the time when legally you will need to have the capability to look after the person with dementia financially. If you plan ahead for this by discussing the role of financial power-of-attorney early you will be prepared when the time comes that the person with dementia is no longer regarded under the law as legally competent to make financial decisions.

Speak to a person who is able to give you advice about financial matters and ensure that you are prepared. In the initial stages, this is best done together so both parties are participating and in agreement about how to proceed. You may need to make changes to legal structures if you own businesses, so that you are both familiar with and can manage the financial arrangements as the condition progresses. You will have enough on your mind without having to manage businesses.

Make sure someone else has copies of important documents so that when one of you dies, the other can be confident that someone knows where everything is located.

It is also important to make a will.

Finger-food

Finger-food is food you can eat on the run, while standing, walking, doing almost anything without sitting down at a table with a knife and fork or spoon. It's food you can eat without utensils – picked up in the fingers, brought to the mouth and eaten.

We are all familiar with the finger-food we are served at social functions. We stand juggling a glass of wine and a plate with a napkin, attempting to eat and drink and talk: chicken wings, small fried pieces, dipping sauces, small sandwiches, party pies

LIVING WITH A PERSON WITH DEMENTIA

and mini sausage rolls. In recent years, the range of finger-food at such events has broadened to include anything you can cut into small pieces, serve on a platter and consume as you stand and talk.

It is an important feature of any dementia care kitbag. Offering finger-food can soothe agitation, interrupt an escalation of distress, or distract a person who is engaging in risky behaviour. It can also help you to provide nutrition when the skills to manage utensils have become lost or inconsistent.

It should be firm enough to hold its shape from the dish or tray to the mouth. An example is cooked broccoli. Florets of broccoli are perfect finger-food. Carrot and celery sticks, small pieces of sausage or other meats can also be finger-food. Essentially, anything that can be held between finger and thumb can be finger-food. You can add herbs and spices or a dipping sauce, depending on the ability of the person with dementia to manage the dipping process. There are recipes on the internet for finger-food for people living with dementia. It may be best to ask friends if they can prepare some finger-foods for you so you have a selection in your fridge or freezer.

Remember the importance of a balanced diet as it can be easy and quick to thaw or heat-up something in the microwave, but do it too often and you may miss out on the nutrition that things like fruit and nuts can provide. Swallowing may also be a problem, so take care to monitor that the person is swallowing successfully. If you are concerned about choking you may need to get a swallowing assessment.

Collect any pieces of food that have been left in the house and provide a hand towel for cleaning up. Check pot-plants! Monitor the person with dementia for weight loss when moving to a finger-food diet as it can happen very quickly.

You may need to think about the entire menu as finger-food. It may be that the person with dementia is unable to manage utensils at all. It may also be that the person does not recognize food as an object anymore. This takes some preparation and thought. You may need to consult a dietitian to ensure that the person you care for is eating a balanced diet. Remember to take medical conditions such as diabetes into account when designing a finger-food menu.

Finger-food is particularly important when a person with dementia becomes agitated or cannot sit for a meal (see *Wandering*).

This means they may be best offered food 'on the run'. Remember hydration as well. This can be a real problem for people with dementia who walk a lot.

A person with dementia will sit and fall asleep if they have a full stomach. This can be the only time the person rests if they have been walking constantly. Keep offering food until they sit or slow down and look as if they might stop walking.

A person with dementia can eat beyond fullness when the usual brain mechanisms that help us recognize fullness fail to work. They can vomit, even as they continue eating. If this occurs more than once, consult a specialist *Behaviour Support Team*. They will help you to respond to this in a holistic way (behavioural strategies and perhaps medication).

Fitness

There is ample research to support the need to maintain your own fitness and that of the person with dementia. Walk together, if you can, at least three times a week. Preferably walk as if you are late, which will get your blood pumping around your brain and body. Evidence suggests that in the brains of mice that exercise, a hormone is released that creates new brain cells. Interesting.

Forgetting

Stephen Post (2000) talks of those with dementia as being 'deeply forgetful'. Forgetting is the hallmark symptom of dementia. It is also the experience of every single human being. We all forget. We need to forget. If we remembered everything we've experienced we would be overloaded with unimportant information and find it very difficult to function. Forgetting serves a useful purpose for us all. However, it becomes a problem when we have difficulty remembering the important information we need to function in daily life.

Forgetting does not take away personhood. It is a specific difficulty. The person remains intact. See *Personhood*.

People with dementia need reminders, gentle reassurance and support to overcome the gaps in memory that increase as the dementia progresses. There are many sources of memory support available through Alzheimer's associations in your country. Make yourself familiar with how to provide support for someone who is 'deeply forgetful'.

One of the basic strategies for countering forgetting is repetition. This is how you learn and how to sustain memories. You can use this with a person with dementia so long as they have the language skills to engage with your verbal prompts. Repeating information enhances memory. It needs to be frequent enough (usually at least daily) and of sufficient interest or importance (salience) to the person that they will make connections to existing information. The more meaningful it is, the more likely they will retain it.

Why am I talking about learning and people with dementia? Because people with dementia can learn. You just have to structure the information so that they can do it.

Friends

Be clear about who are the friends of the person with dementia so you can contact them to engage them and encourage them to visit the person you care for and be involved socially. They may need some encouragement to stay in touch. It is very important that they do keep in contact for as long as they can as social engagement stimulates memory and mood. Relationships are vital for well-being.

Gardening

The benefits of gardening are well known. If you have a garden and the person with dementia has enjoyed gardening in the past, it may continue to be a source of pleasure and satisfaction. Sunshine is vital for Vitamin D production. There are physical benefits to all the activities involved in gardening. There is pleasure in planting, smelling and tasting plants (not all plants – be clear which are okay to eat!), and harvesting the produce of your vegetable garden.

However, you may find that maintaining a garden (vegetables particularly) takes too much of your time and planning to be practical anymore. If that is the case, take up visiting community gardens and public botanical gardens. This is a great seasonal activity that provides enjoyment and opportunities for socializing that are not totally dependent on you making it happen.

You could decide to focus on a few pots and engage in planting activities together. Be aware that planting and pulling-out may become mixed up for the person with dementia. Be prepared to replant as necessary and don't get too invested in the plants growing. You may need to visit a big-box store or plant nursery to top up or replace plants that have been pulled out while the person you care for was walking around the garden yesterday.

Wash hands after gardening. Although you may remember to do it the person you care for may not. Be prepared to remind them gently: 'We'll have to wash our hands now.' Model it for them.

Gestures

Communication involves more than words. It involves gestures. This is a form of body language that enhances the messages you communicate. Be clear in your gestures. You may need to make sure the person is looking at you so they pick up the message of the gesture.

Examples of gestures include palms up and fingers out to the person (usually indicates a receptive approach); fist (anger); pointed finger (blame); palms out, fingers upward (stop); hands up, palms facing to you, fingers moving toward you repeatedly (invitation). You usually make verbal statements to accompany these gestures. This enhances comprehension.

Going out

Socializing and shopping are opportunities for contact with others. This creates well-being. The skills of social behaviour and shopping can enhance well-being. There will come a point in your excursion where mixing socially or in shopping centres or shops in general becomes too stressful or confusing. When you see signs of confusion or reluctance it is time to return to the quiet and familiarity of home.

Prepare yourself for your journey out by thinking about the level of stimulation you will both encounter; the clothes you and the person with dementia will need; whether you will eat when

LIVING WITH A PERSON WITH DEMENTIA

out; whether the person you care for will need the toilet; and how familiar with dementia the people you will encounter are when out. This preparation is important but takes some practice to get right. You learn from each journey out. You may find that among other things you need a backpack with a change of clothes. Be prepared for all events.

Guardianship

The laws of guardianship are different in each country, so familiarize yourself with your local laws. Guardianship is the role taken by a person appointed legally to take over responsibility for someone when they can no longer take responsibility for themselves – when they are no longer legally 'competent'.

As dementia progresses there will come a point where you or another person may be appointed guardian for the person you care for. It is important that you are familiar with the nature of this responsibility. There are legal obligations and limitations and you must fulfil your role according to your local laws.

Guilt

See also *Burnout, Respite*

Guilt is a common experience for caregivers when they take time for themselves. Guilt is a normal human emotion that tells you when you have hurt someone by doing something or by not doing something, by thinking something that is morally wrong even though you have not actually done it.

Even planning *respite* can make some caregivers feel guilty. Some find the guilty feeling so painful that they avoid taking time off at all. Consequently, they can become exhausted and overwhelmed and have to stop caregiving for a period of time. *Burnout* can be a real problem for caregivers who are driven from within themselves to maintain unrealistic levels of caregiving, often to avoid the guilt that arises when they do anything to care for themselves.

It is as if being a caregiver means always giving care and never caring for yourself; as if to care for yourself is selfish. The next step in this process is to feel guilty just because you wanted a rest, a break or a morning off to have coffee with a friend, or even a couple of hours to go to the doctor for yourself.

If you are to survive as a caregiver and be there for the long haul of years as a dementia caregiver, you are going to have to deal with guilt. You must find a way to overcome it so that you can care for yourself. This is essential or you simply won't be a caregiver for as long as you want to be. You will burn out.

How to deal with guilt? It's a feeling that you have done something wrong. It is not the reality. Sometimes feelings do not give us good information about reality. This is one of those times. You actually have not done anything wrong. It is just a feeling. All you have done is plan a holiday, or take a morning off to see a friend, or taken a week to recuperate so you can come back refreshed. That is not wrong. If this approach isn't enough to get you to take some time for yourself because of guilt, you may need to see a therapist to get you over the line. However, that may provoke guilt too!

Hallucinations

These are false sensory experiences. They are often confused with *delusions*, which are fixed false ideas. Hallucinations can be experienced in any sensory modality. They are a common experience in psychosis, which can occur at any age. Psychosis is a common experience in dementia as the brain undergoes changes from normal function.

Visual hallucinations involve 'seeing things' that are not there. It may be little people on the curtain rail that appear every night and carry on conversations with the person. I once knew a woman who lived on her own and the little people provided her with company in the evening. Her mind cleverly created a way for her to have companionship in an otherwise solitary life.

Auditory hallucinations are commonly referred to as 'hearing things' or 'hearing voices'. People with auditory hallucinations often report hearing a voice commanding them to do something, telling them to be wary of people they should not trust, or a voice making derogatory statements about themselves. These can be distressing.

Tactile hallucinations are false touch experiences and may consist of sensing bugs under the skin which cause the person to scratch their skin badly.

Gustatory hallucinations are false taste experiences. This may include a taste of faeces, or metal, or any other common taste in the absence of food.

Olfactory hallucinations are false experiences of smell, odour or aroma. People with dementia may report smelling any common aroma despite it not being present.

Hallucinations are often a cause of worry for caregivers and other family members. Just hallucinating, however, is not a cause for concern. The major reason hallucinations become a cause for concern is if the person is distressed or their daily functioning is affected (for example, if they refuse to leave the house for fear of encountering people they see or if displeased voices tell them to stay home).

The best approach, as with many experiences the person with dementia may report, is to not dispute or challenge it. Be curious. Ask questions but avoid 'Why?', as this can be perceived as a challenge. Avoid arguing about whether it is real or not. A dispute or challenge will only create ill-feeling and cause the person with dementia to either withdraw or become angry and/or aggressive.

Validate the experience by asking questions so you can understand more about what they are experiencing. Your primary goal here is to work out what their experience and perception are and then offer a response. How are they affected emotionally? This will give you a clue as to how to respond – for example, if they are angry (people become angry when they are afraid or feel disrespected), you could reassure them; if they are sad/distressed, comfort, reassure or distract them.

Questions to ask include: 'Tell me what you are seeing/hearing/feeling so I can understand', or engage in a discussion about what to do about the voice or vision: 'Well, what do you think we could do about it? What else could you do, other than remain at home? Is there another solution? Maybe we could go out together, rather than you walk on your own. Would that work?' Reassure the person that they are safe with you and that you will protect them. If this doesn't calm them you may need to leave where you are if the location is part of the problem; for example, the people they can hear may be dead family members who used to live in the house. Go for a drive and a coffee before returning. As a last resort you may need to consult a medical professional and use medication as prescribed to assist in calming the person. This should always follow other efforts to calm them.

Happiness

This is a fleeting experience that influencers on Instagram want to sell by the bottle. Good luck with that. Contentment is a more lasting experience to strive for.

Happiness comes and goes and is not the goal. It is a by-product of doing what we find meaningful and enjoyable. People with dementia can experience these moments of happiness as much as any of us can. So long as you provide opportunities for such pleasure, happiness will be a part of it.

So, don't go for happiness. Go for contentment.

Health

There are four pillars of good health: good sleep, good food, exercise and social engagement.

Your need for sleep changes through your life. Adapt the amount of sleep you aim for to what your body tells you. It will fluctuate from night to night. The best indicator of how much sleep you need is your tiredness during the day. Sleep may be disrupted when you are caring for a person with dementia. If so, try to organize some overnight respite care so you can get periods of uninterrupted sleep.

Good food means don't skimp on food by eating mostly fast-food or toast. Make time in your caregiving day to do meal preparation, together if possible. Engage the person with dementia in as much of this activity as you can. Maintain a balanced diet, particularly if the person is no longer able to sit for an entire meal and is moving to a finger-food diet. This requires monitoring how much the person actually ingests, not just how much you offer or prepare, as they may take it from you but put it down somewhere in the house and not actually eat it.

Exercise is critical for good health for you and the person you

LIVING WITH A PERSON WITH DEMENTIA

care for. It helps maintain brain function and has been explored in the section *Exercise*.

The fourth pillar of good health is social engagement. We are social beings. We are made for relationships with others, and as a caregiver you may find that your social life has shrunk since you began your caregiving role. One of the most severe problems facing caregivers is social isolation. It is just you and the person you care for and there doesn't seem to be room for anyone else in your world any more. This can be a slippery slope to burnout. Respite care is essential. In other words, organize breaks so you can catch up with friends, family or support groups. Make it a priority. Your health and your longevity as a caregiver depend on it. If you try to be heroic you will likely 'crash and burn' much sooner than you need to.

Hearing

Being hard of hearing or deaf can make it difficult to feel part of conversations. It may cause a person to lose confidence and want to avoid social settings that are noisy. There is some research to suggest that hearing difficulties are associated with increased risk of dementia. As a caregiver, ensure that hearing aids are charged, clean and ready for use. You may also need to make an appointment for the person with dementia to have an annual hearing test to ensure the hearing aids are up to date.

If the person you care for has a hearing problem, when it comes to social situations there are some things you can do to help them hear better. Ensure that they are sitting with their back to a wall so they are not surrounded by noise. Choose quiet cafes. When talking to them, look at them so they can make the most of visual and auditory cues. For more help, consult your local deaf association.

Helplessness

Helplessness can become a problem if the person with dementia adopts a position of relying too much on you for things they can do themselves. This means they have given up trying and it can result in under-use of their intact skills and knowledge. This may be a problem for them in the long term as the maintenance of skills and knowledge relies on engaging in daily challenges such as dressing, eating and self-care. Helplessness will cause them to decline more quickly.

The person must be encouraged and supported to maintain their abilities by doing what they can do. This requires effort on your part and you may have to search around to find the key that gets them to engage with tasks and not rely on you for everything. A healthy approach is for them to rely on you for what they cannot do and for you to be willing to provide that much and no more.

Hitting

Hitting is a form of physical *aggression* that usually occurs in response to rising feelings of *anger* that the person cannot contain. It is a signal to stop what you are doing and make yourself safe by standing out of reach. It is a response. It does not occur in a vacuum.

Identify the cause. The cause is the 'A' of the ABC behaviour model discussed in Part I of this book. There may be multiple causes. Is there something in the environment contributing to the hitting? Is it due to something you have done or not done? Is it within the person, for example pain?

Hitting often occurs when you are in close proximity to the person and usually during personal care. Ask yourself what the person with dementia seems to be making of your presence. Are they frustrated because you are doing too much, doing it too quickly, or being too patronizing in your tone, or have they misunderstood your presence and perceive you as intruding in their private space having forgotten who you are? Are you chatting too much and it is annoying them?

If the cause is environmental, it may be too much noise. If so, turn the music off or ask people in the house to quieten down. If the room is too hot, open a window or turn on a fan, or change clothing to be suitable for the weather.

Hobbies

Keep up the interests of the person with dementia as much as possible. This helps promote and support memory, skills and knowledge. For instance, if the person is a woodworker, they may be able to continue doing projects adapted to their memory and physical abilities. It may be that they can still visit the woodworking club and workshop and participate in projects with the support of some of the members who are able to adjust and scaffold the tasks so the person you care for can continue to participate and have experiences of success. This can promote a feeling of belonging and identity.

Also keep up your own interests as much as possible by organizing regular respite breaks or weekly support.

Holding

This is not physical holding but psychological holding. To be held is to feel secure and safe. Your role as caregiver is to psychologically hold or help the person with dementia feel secure and safe. You may psychologically hold the person with dementia by validating them, by reminding them of something about themselves that brings a feeling of comfort and pleasure – or it may be offering them an object or food that you know brings focus and calm.

Home

Home is an experience we each have that may be related to a place or people. It may be a feeling of safety and contentment or it may mean memories of stress and uncertainty. As dementia progresses, the person you care for may look for a home they once experienced when they were children. Even if it was a place of stress, the familiarity it offers may prompt them to search for it or desire it. Photos of past houses they lived in or of their parents or siblings may activate memories that calm them. Such prompts for reminiscence can be a helpful tool to have readily at hand. Other prompts may include objects or keepsakes that they associate with home, either currently or from past periods of their life.

Hope

Holding hope for the person with dementia is an important role for the caregiver. Be hopeful that they can experience joy, moments of happiness and pleasure, that they can recover from upset, that they can manage some things but not others, that they can cope with some stresses and not others, that they can manage some situations safely, and can thrive if provided with opportunities for risk-taking. Giving up hope leads to fearfully taking control and despairing for them. This ultimately leads to misery for them and for you.

Housework

Some domestic tasks are necessary for maintenance and cleanliness of your home. The person with dementia may benefit from actively participating in these tasks. They may be able to sweep, set the table, replace cutlery and crockery in cupboards or drawers, take plates to the sink, tidy items in the house. Such responsibilities can provide a sense of importance and value. You may need to label cupboards and drawers so they can find the right location if they have forgotten. You may also have to become accepting of finding the knives in the cupboard and the cups in the fridge. If you modify the task to what you know they can succeed at, domestic tasks can be a source of well-being for the person you care for.

Hugging

Hugs are usually a source of comfort and an expression of emotional closeness. They can be an opportunity for the person with dementia to be held with affection, without it necessarily becoming sexual. Regular hugs throughout the day can be a way to punctuate the activity of the day with moments of resting in close contact.

If you or the person with dementia are not comfortable with physical contact, hugs may be a source of discomfort. You may have to modify your own reactions in order to match the needs of the person with dementia. If they are showing a reluctance to hug you may have to resist the urge to hug them. Stroking or simply touching on the arm and making eye contact may be all the closeness they can tolerate. Match your actions to what they can manage and look for signs of well-being, enjoyment and peace or contentment with the touch.

Humour

A good sense of humour is not only useful when dating online ('must have GSOH'), it is also valuable in caregivers for people with dementia when confronted with hilarious or difficult situations. If your partner comes to breakfast with his underwear over his trousers ready to go shopping you may need your sense of humour and some patience.

For people with dementia, humour may be difficult to find and not just because life can be difficult for them. Neurologically, humour requires you to be able to see another side of a situation or an alternative meaning to words. This may not be possible if the frontal lobes are depleted due to dementia. Frontal lobes help you to shift perspective. Frontal lobe impairment affects humour by diminishing the ability to shift perspective and connect with unrelated information. It may also be that the person has become rather concrete and literal in their interpretation of a joke or situation and so flippant comments can be interpreted as hurtful. Be alert to signs that they are not 'getting' the joke. They may not be able to see the funny side of it. Try it and back off if it doesn't work.

If the person with dementia still has a capacity for humour a good laugh together can relieve tension and cement rapport.

Hunger

Hunger is the internal signal that we need to eat. We can usually manage our response to the urge to eat and decide not to eat or to prepare a meal. Hunger can be stimulated by smells and the sight of food cooking, by remembering we have not eaten for some time, or by the sensation we get when our stomach grumbles, or by the pre-meal routine of table setting and washing hands. Any of these causes may be enough to stimulate the person to eat.

However, hunger can become a problem if there is no 'off-switch' or experience of fullness. Some people with dementia may

A-Z OF DEMENTIA CARE AT HOME

not recognize the sensation of fullness. This can lead to *overeating*, which can have a drastic impact on weight gain and other associated health problems such as diabetes if the overeating involves sweet drinks, and so on. As a caregiver, you may need to monitor the availability of food or the types of food kept in the house.

The fridge can become an attractive source of food for the person. If this occurs, you may need to restrict access with a child-safe device.

Hygiene

This topic is covered extensively in *Bathing, Assault, Negotiation, Privacy*, and in the Part I discussion of consequences.

Personal care is something you do each day for yourself in private. But when dementia robs you of the skills to do this as independently and reliably as before, you need help to do it. Good hygiene is essential for socializing and for your own sense of dignity and identity. As a caregiver, you will be required to help maintain the person's hygiene and this may be a challenging part of dementia care for you. It may be helpful to have discussions with other caregivers and with support organizations that specialize in this so that all of it does not fall to you and you are prepared for it when the time comes.

Identity

Knowing who you are is an early life experience that comes with the onset of language acquisition. 'I am...' It gives you a way to introduce yourself to others, and a confidence that you can be with others, with a sense of yourself. Over the journey of life your identity may have been positive and healthy or it may have been insecure and riven with anxieties about whether you were as good as others, could hold a place with others.

Personal identity develops through life as you gain a job/career, take up roles of parent and grandparent, neighbour, volunteer, leader. As dementia progresses, many of these involvements recede and disappear from daily life, leaving a hole that can result in a depressive withdrawal. It can also cause the person to search for ways to find a sense of identity by engaging in

LIVING WITH A PERSON WITH DEMENTIA

previously valued activities. This may now be unsafe or leave the person open to rejection or criticism that can come from making social mistakes. Your role as a caregiver can be to pave the way by preparing people for the person with dementia so that they can be accepted and valued with positive feedback and encouragement or reassurance.

Identity is not just knowing who you are and being able to remember your name. It is also affirmed and given to you by how others treat you, behave towards you, speak to you. The person with dementia may experience being spoken to as if they are a child. This can often diminish a person and is referred to as 'dementia speak' or infantilization.

Identity enables you to be connected to others and to find a place in society, to have a sense of your value. As dementia progresses and social roles are diminished, *attachments* and *comfort* become more and more important for maintaining well-being. In other words, how the person is able to connect to you and others with affection, affirmation and recognition will matter more and more in helping them feel like their old self.

Ignoring

Being ignored leads to isolation and disempowerment. People with dementia are frequently ignored in social settings where verbal fluency and agile memory are taken for granted. As a caregiver, you can make a difference. You can do it by making a concerted effort to ensure that the person with dementia is included by reminding others in your circle to include them, to make eye contact, to invite them, to ask appropriate questions, to support them with accurately tailored help.

Ill-being

Ill-being is a word coined by Tom Kitwood (1997) to capture the negative experience that is the opposite of well-being. It includes such actions as *ignoring, infantilization, disempowerment* and *imposition.*

The signs that a person is in a state of ill-being include: negative mood (shows tension and upset in facial expression, posture and sounds, such as whimpering, calling out, screaming or crying), depressed, grieving, sad, angry, aggressive, agitated or restless, anxiety or fear, boredom, bodily tension, easily dominated by others, rejected or ignored by others, listlessness, apathy, withdrawal, physical discomfort or pain, unable to enjoy things, lonely, makes noise, calls out or vocalizes, verbally refuses care, suspicious of others, and physically threatens others.

Illness

People with dementia may not be able to communicate being ill as easily as you can. This may be because of not perceiving the experience or not having the words to tell you about it. Experiences of pain may not make sense to the person and may cause confusion and irritability but not be expressed by them as 'I am in pain'.

As a caregiver, you have to be a detective who notices small changes in demeanour and mood. The list of signs of ill-being are a good starting point. Watch for indicators of pain and discomfort, for changes in behaviour and appearance that signal that something is not right. Then act as appropriate.

Implicit memory

This is a type of memory that you are not aware of. It is often referred to as automatic or unconscious memory. It is the memory you have for complex activities such as dressing, driving a car, talking fluently, approaching a social setting and extending your hand in greeting. How do you know how to do that? It is so well learned that it is automatic and you do not have to think about it. Same for dressing. You just know that you put your underwear on first and then your other clothing and finally a jumper or coat and tie.

However, as dementia progresses these automatic sequences of action that are so well learned and not thought about gradually degrade so that you need assistance to complete previously automatic tasks. It becomes effortful to get dressed, to remember how to eat, how to put a sentence together, how to make social connections.

As these skills are lost, the job of a caregiver is to scaffold the experience, to be the Sherpa who provides just enough support, structure and information to ensure success. You could say you are successful if the person with dementia doesn't notice you are doing it.

The person with dementia can become frustrated and despondent because implicit memory has failed them. It is useful in these situations for you to provide encouragement and support that is just enough to help them get back on track and find small successes because of your scaffolding.

Imposition

Imposition occurs when we impose our own desires or priorities or will on another person. With people who have dementia, imposition is all too common. It may be a simple act of deciding what they will wear today, when they have the capacity to make that decision themselves. It may be deciding to cut up their food for them without asking when they may have the capacity to do it themselves or at least to tell you what they want to occur.

Imposition is harmful because it robs people with dementia of the opportunity to exercise agency, skills and knowledge. It ultimately creates *excess disability* and hastens the progress of dementia.

Inclusion

Social inclusion is important to most of us for a satisfying life. It can be on a grand scale of inclusion of people in particular groups. And it can be on a micro scale of being included in a conversation. People with dementia are at risk of being excluded, often not out of malice but out of lack of awareness of their need for social support to maintain inclusion and participation in social acts of conversation, decision-making, planning and choices. Exclusion is painful and results in ill-being and excess disability.

As a caregiver your role is to scaffold the person's presence and inclusion by raising awareness, by prompting others and by advocating for the person. This may mean interrupting the flow of a conversation to include the person you care for so that they can participate as an equal and so the others can rise to the occasion and make changes to the way they communicate.

Incontinence

Incontinence occurs more frequently in dementia as the person is not alerted to the cues for using their bladder or bowel or misinterprets the physical sensations. This topic is explored elsewhere in detail.

See *Continence, Bedwetting, Soiling.*

Independence

Dementia can challenge independence and make it difficult to maintain the abilities that we once took for granted.

The role of a caregiver is to support and enable, encouraging and facilitating as much independence as possible. Your job is to scaffold life so the person with dementia can be as independent as possible. This will change as the effects of dementia progress. You may find yourself having to do more to support personal care or social interaction. You may find that as the condition advances your role becomes more one of providing affection and physical comfort than social engagement or activities. Be alert to the actual needs of the person as they shift and change.

Indifference

This is akin to *apathy, passivity* and the *lack of motivation* that characterizes frontal lobe impairment. The person may seem as though they are depressed. However, it may be due to the neurological changes that mimic depression rather than actual low mood. Their mood might be fine but you won't know that until you provide the stimulus to activate them. It may be that the indifference they experience is too profound for your stimulus and they remain indifferent. You may have to cast around and discuss the problem with your support group or person. You may need to choose your time for activating them and leave them alone at other times. Otherwise, you may find yourself knocking your head against the brick wall of their indifference. Choose your moments and make it matter; for example, to get them out for a walk may require half an hour of preparation and encouragement. Put some thought into how you will do this and have options in mind if one approach does not work. You will be providing the motivation that they lack.

Infantilization

Speaking to, or in other ways treating, a person as if they were a child is infantilization. Examples include using a sing-song tone of voice that is often heard with childcare workers. It may be telling the person off as a punitive parent might do: 'Oh, look what a mess you've made. Here, let me do it.' Or: 'No, you can't do that. You'll only hurt yourself.' Or reminding the person of past problems: 'Careful darling, you know you have trouble with pasta. Let me do that for you.'

In this last instance, infantilization is combined with imposition to diminish the person's skills and prevent food falling from the utensil. This may be more of a worry for the anxious caregiver than for the person with dementia. As a caregiver, your job is to relax enough to let the mess happen. The priority is the independence and emotional well-being of the person with dementia. Get hold of your anxiety and manage it long enough for the person to eat their meal. Clean up afterwards with as little fuss as possible and no mention of it to the person. They have likely done their best. What is the point of telling them off? Usually it's just to discharge your own frustration.

Insomnia

Difficulty sleeping or a disrupted sleep-wake cycle can occur in anyone's life. In dementia, it is believed to occur because of changes to the levels of neurotransmitters that regulate the sleep-wake cycle. The cues for sleep are light and dark and the feeling of tiredness. The person with dementia may not be 'reading the signals' as reliably as they once did, causing them to disconnect from night-time and daytime rhythms.

One way to respond to this is to orient the person. Show them it is dark outside. Another is to change into nightwear yourself. This signals readiness for bed. Preparation for bedtime may also include a hot drink and quiet time with all screens switched off (including the TV).

Sometimes you may find that the person with dementia wants to engage in nocturnal activity as if it is daytime. You may be able to re-orient them to the time of day by doing some of the suggestions mentioned. However, if that is not effective, it may be best to go along with it and participate in what they want to do. The main purpose of your presence is to ensure their safety – for example, so that they do not leave the house – and provide some companionship if it is needed.

Intact abilities

Use it or lose it. Even though some abilities are diminished or lost over the progress of the dementia, other abilities will remain intact. As a companion carer you can help the person to remain as active and engaged as possible at each step along the way by scaffolding their experience, supporting practice and success. Each success keeps the remaining skills and knowledge active and intact.

Intimacy

This refers to emotional closeness. Sexual intimacy is addressed elsewhere (see *Sex*).

Emotional closeness remains possible for many people with dementia and their intimates (partner or friends) well into the dementia. This form of intimacy relies on the ability to express one's need for comfort and affection. It does not need words or rational explanation or logic.

It can be sitting quietly on a couch together, perhaps holding hands, perhaps not, aware of each other's presence, not having to say anything but comfortable and content. The person with dementia may express a need for this type of closeness well into the more advanced periods of the dementia when words have long failed them. You do not need words to be emotionally close.

In fact, as words diminish in importance, non-verbal ways of expressing intimacy become more important.

Intimidation

This is a form of bullying that is used by people to get another person to do what they want. It may consist of raising your voice, using your facial expression, your posture or gestures such as a raised fist, or it may be physical contact such as a push or hit. It is not okay to engage in intimidation with people with dementia, no matter how frustrated you are.

It creates fear, anger and perhaps compliance, but it also creates withdrawal, loss of trust, and resentment. Quality of life drops for both parties when intimidation is used to gain compliance.

Invalidation

Invalidation is the effect of having someone deny your reality, desires or intention and impose their reality or priorities on you. It treats your perspective as worthless. Examples of invalidation include: 'Don't cry', 'You're not hungry', 'You're just being selfish', 'You don't want to wear those trousers/that dress'.

Being on the receiving end of invalidation is one of the most disabling experiences you can have as a human being. It crushes confidence in one's own perspective and judgement, and increases self-doubt. People with dementia make mistakes. We all do. But the confidence to 'have a go' can be diminished if you are constantly dominated and invalidated by the people whose role it is to care for you.

Jokes

See *Humour*

Joy

To enjoy is to 'be in joy'. Joy is underestimated. It is a positive emotional experience that lifts us up and makes us feel good about life, move closer to others and be more generous and kind. What gives you joy? What gives the person you care for joy? Is it music? Dancing? Is it doing something they have loved all their life, such as visiting the theatre or ballet? Or perhaps it is bush-walking/rambling? As a caregiver, look for opportunities for joy.

Think about the ways the person you care for enjoyed life in the past, before dementia. It could be visiting their former place of employment, or a former sports club, or doing a hobby they gave their lives to over decades but which is no longer possible. A friend was a woodworker for all his adult life until dementia made it difficult for him to continue to participate. A visit to a local woodwork group workshop that had large machinery, hand tools and benches calmed him and gave him pleasure as he walked slowly up to the benches and stroked the timber, held the tools and put them down. He 'talked wood' and furniture making to the woodworkers who spoke with him and encouraged him to touch their work. This gave him joy.

Labelling

Labels are poisonous to self-esteem. We use them in everyday life because they provide a short-hand way of talking about others. But they reduce unique people to stereotypes and we lose individuality. We lose the person.

Labels that can be common in dementia care include: 'He's a wanderer', 'He's aggressive', 'He's a fall risk', 'He's manipulative', 'He's attention-seeking', 'He's lazy', 'He's a full-feed', 'He's a shower', 'He's a full assist'.

Avoid them by using descriptive, non-labelling terms: 'She likes to walk a lot', 'He can be aggressive when he is afraid', 'He can fall over if he is tired', 'He has difficulty being straightforward about what he wants', 'He needs your attention regularly', 'He needs a prompt to get going', 'He needs your help to eat', 'He needs full assistance with personal care'.

Language

See *Infantilization*, *Labelling*

Laughter

My three-year-old granddaughter has the best cackle when she realizes her intention to spread honey on the table has been seen and she hurries to do it before I can get to her. She is a happy girl and moments of laughter punctuate our time with her. She trusts me and my wife, and knows she is accepted and safe.

Laughter releases hormones that make us feel good, lighter and happier. It is an effective antidepressant with no bad side-effects. I am hard of hearing. The times I mis-hear what my wife has said to me often cause us to laugh at the silliness of what I thought she said.

Dementia care can be hard work and frustrating. You need moments of laughter to break up the stressful moments and punctuate life with lightness. There will be many moments when the ridiculous nature of life and what we do or say occurs to you and you see the funny side of life. If you start laughing it is possible the person you care for will also start laughing. Not laughing at but laughing with.

Learning

People with dementia can learn. Sounds obvious but it is only in the last few decades that this has become accepted. Previously it was thought that people with dementia are unable to learn and so you should not waste your time trying to teach them anything new or ask them to adapt or adjust. If you adjust and adapt to their needs and capacities as they change through the process of dementia you can be successful.

Repetition is important so that you work within the limits of short-term memory. Make what you are trying to teach the person salient or relevant or interesting to them. If it is meaningful they will remember it better. Associate it with something already well learned. These are the basics. Follow these and you will have success helping people with dementia to learn.

Leaving home

See *Unsafe leaving*

Lewy body disease (LBD)

Lewy body disease is the third most common cause of dementia. It is characterized by fluctuating or unpredictable changes in alertness and attention, mood, thinking and behaviour. Visual hallucinations and difficulty with movement, particularly walking, all occur in a pattern of progressive decline.

The Lewy bodies are clumps of protein that occur in areas of the brain that affect thinking, movement and memory. The symptoms are often mistaken for Parkinson's disease and so early diagnosis and treatment are important. The onset can be earlier than is usual for other dementias such as Alzheimer's dementia. And the progress can be quicker. Diagnosis and a treatment plan are important to help guide everyone involved.

Life story

A person's life story influences their personality, memories, defences and daily choices. That is true for the person with dementia and for you. Early parenting, family of origin, trauma, loving relationships, education, employment history, friendships, hobbies, war experience, all go to make up the person's internal narrative, self-identity, defences and emotional and social preferences. If you understand where the person has come from, you can adjust and enhance your activity with them.

Knowing the person's life story can help you in moments of stress. Perhaps you are assisting the person to shower or to dress and they become confused or overwhelmed. You can prompt recall of an aspect of their life story by asking questions that activate memory. An example may be: 'Tom, you were a boilermaker, weren't you? What does a boilermaker do? Was it dangerous? What did you have to wear? Did you have good friends at work?'

Avoid questions about wartime experience unless you know the person well and are sure that the person doesn't mind talking about it. Wartime memories can often be filled with regrets if they have killed people, or trauma from what they have done, seen or heard, or not done. However, be ready to talk about wartime if the person wakes at night with a wartime nightmare or is walking about the house concerned that the enemy is trying to break in.

It can also be an opportunity to talk about respect and admiration for war service. It may take the form of sitting with the person to go through old photographs. Or it may be a life-story book that you or family members have put together. This can consist of photographs or copies of photographs and a brief paragraph explaining each one that tells the story of the person's life. This life-story book can be available to every caregiver who comes into the house. It can also be available to the person with dementia to go through on their own at times of negative feeling or disturbance and it can become a 'touchstone' as it were, that the person goes to in times of need. Leave it out on the table.

This book is an aid to memory that activates and maintains the person's story in their own mind. By prompting the person's recall of events, you can create moments of pleasure and contentment and overcome building agitation and restlessness. If you reconnect to your story, you can often feel calmer and more peaceful.

It takes some time to put a life-story book together but it is worth the effort.

Light

Light is a vital component of life. For people with dementia whose lives can become dysregulated, light is important to regulate their sleep-wake cycle and mood. Ensure the person has access to light through the daylight hours by spending some time outdoors. This is also good for sustaining Vitamin D levels as light on skin activates the production of Vitamin D, which is vital for bone strength.

The sleep-wake cycle can become disrupted if the person with dementia is sleeping into the daylight hours. It is possible to shift the sleep-wake cycle to regular day-night by waking the person at an earlier time and giving them exposure to sunlight.

Mood is also affected by light or the absence of it. Some people are more susceptible to the effects of light than others. If this is a factor for the person you care for you may need to ensure the person has regular exposure to sunlight. Also observe how bright the lights are in your house. Do you need to increase their brightness?

Likes/dislikes

We all have personal preferences. In some sense they make us who we are. In a person-centred approach to caregiving, these are a vital piece of information for you to know how to respond to the person. Find out what they like and dislike so you can meet these needs in the same way you hope someone might do for you.

Limit setting

Setting limits is a well-known behavioural strategy for shaping a person's behaviour. It is used with children and with adults. Often it is used in everyday interactions without you recognizing that that is what you are doing.

Limit setting with people with dementia is useful but must be done in a way that is kind and aimed to enhance the person's experience, such as making them safer. Examples of limits include: 'You can't go outside. It's raining', 'Please eat one mouthful at a time', 'Two scones, Mavis', 'It's time to go to bed', 'You've had sex with me once today. That's enough. Let's have a cuddle in bed and go to sleep.'

It matters how the limit is stated. It must be done in a neutral, non-punishing tone. If you are angry or frustrated, the limit may come across as a punishment. Try to take the anger out of your voice before you state the limit. If the person thinks they are being punished, this can generate an angry resentful reaction, rather than the desired compliance.

Listening, active

Active listening is a set of skills that can improve your communication with the person with dementia.

Communication is essentially expressing and comprehending (understanding). In order to do these two things, we need to listen actively. We often assume we listen well but most of the time we listen in order to interrupt with our own thoughts rather than listen to understand.

Active listening involves a conscious effort to be attentive, to be aware that the person is trying to communicate with you right now and needs you to understand. Use eye contact if appropriate. Avoid staring at the person but make sure they know they have your attention by actually looking at them. Stop whatever else you are doing and focus on them. If you continue to mop the floor while they are talking, the message you convey to them with your body language is: 'You are not as important to me as my clean floor.'

It also means you don't judge what you hear but listen to the end and don't interrupt.

Think about what you have heard for a moment. Think about what it means or what the person communicates to you. What do they want you to understand from this? What do they need right now? What does this mean? Think about how the person feels right now. What feelings do they want you to understand? Use your empathy to gain a sense of what they want or need from you in this moment.

Next clarify with questions so you make sure you understand accurately. 'Can you help me understand? Did you mean...?' or 'Do you want the...?'

You can also ask open questions. These are questions of how, what, when, where, who and why. These questions seek more information than a closed question that requires only a yes or no answer, such as 'Did you clean your teeth?'

Respond to the feeling content if it is prominent: 'I'm sorry this has worried you so much.' Then act to remedy or address the concern the person has. If you listen and do nothing, the person may feel more powerless, isolated and hopeless. Active listening is a way to connect, to sustain or build a bond of common understanding and purpose. From an attachment point of view, it is a way to ensure that healthy attachments are sustained.

Listen with your soul.

Greg and Irene have been married for 52 years. Irene has been caring for Greg who has had dementia for the past four years. He is no longer able to use words. One evening Irene is watching TV when she smells faeces. She walks to the lounge door and in the passage Greg is standing fully dressed with faeces over his hands and smeared over his face and hair. She is horrified and lets out, 'Oh no, what have you done!?' She stops and realizes he is telling her something he cannot say in words. She feels sure he is telling her he feels like shit and needs her help. He stood there in front of her and she said, 'Wait there my love and I will be back.' She returns with a towel and disposable wipes. She takes his hand and says, 'What about a shower, my love?' She undresses him gently, talking all the while, smiling and looking at him, letting him know that she wants to connect with him and accepts him, loves him. Once he is dressed again in pyjamas, ready for bed, she cleans up the bedroom where he had defecated. That night she holds him in bed and he sleeps quietly for the first time in many nights.

Long-term memory

See also *Short-term memory*, *Forgetting*

This is the memory for past events, people and experiences. It is located deep within the temporal lobe, in the inner layers of the hippocampus, an area of the brain responsible for memory.

In dementia, long-term memory is more reliable than short-term memory. As the condition progresses, past events can be recalled with considerable detail for longer than more recent events. What happened in the person's childhood will likely be more vivid and more easily recalled than what happened yesterday or this morning.

Life-story books and conversations about the past rely on the recall of long-term memory. It can be worthwhile utilizing this feature of memory in your daily caregiving as it connects the person with their past and their identity and potentially creates positive feeling. Just the act of successfully remembering something can be a positive experience for the person with dementia.

This can be useful as you can assist the person to bring to mind events or relationships with people from the past if you know that these memories are connected to positive feelings. You can also avoid certain topics that you know cause negative or unpleasant memories.

Love, affection

See also *Hugging*

Love is one of the emotions that enables us to connect and sustain relationships with others. Some people can have loving feelings for many people, some for a few. For people with dementia, this is no different. Feeling positively and warmly towards another person enhances our well-being and the well-being of others. These positive feelings may be expressed in many ways, including hugging, kissing and holding hands.

As adults, we tend to become more settled in our relationships and not engage in open demonstrations of affection, particularly in public. However, some people with dementia may be more open and expressive of their affectionate and loving feelings than they were in the past. This can be overwhelming or unnerving for some people. However, as a caregiver, if you prepare others for it, they can be calmer and receive these expressions of love warmly and openly. If they are not prepared for it, they may reject these expressions or be tense and cause the person with dementia to feel uncertain and a sense of having made a mistake.

Lying

Lying usually occurs in an attempt to protect yourself by hiding the truth. If the truth is discovered, you may fear being hurt, rejected or excluded, and feeling ashamed. Everyone does it from time to time. You modify the truth so that someone will not be angry or sad.

A person with dementia may lie for any of the above reasons and it will usually be consistent with their personality. For example, a person with dementia may have always been sensitive to making mistakes and sought to hide their errors from others to avoid feeling ashamed of getting things wrong. They will likely continue to try to hide their forgetfulness or other mistakes, which are likely to become more frequent.

The best response you can make as a caregiver is to ignore the mistakes, forgetfulness or whatever else the person does that causes them to feel ashamed. The only time a mistake needs to be brought to their attention is when it causes a risk to physical safety. All else can be let go.

The purpose of lying is to protect the self from a perceived attack. Do not argue with or accuse the person with dementia of lying. Affirm the person for success and that they are a good and valuable person regardless of how they act.

Malignant social psychology

This term was originally coined by Professor Tom Kitwood in 1997 to refer to the culture of harmful and negative treatment of people with dementia that has a damaging toxic effect on them. His purpose was to highlight the damaging effects of a culture of caregiving that was paternalistic and patronizing, that treated people as children, that ignored people as feeling beings and treated them as less than fully human.

He identified ways this is done and several of these have been examined throughout this book (*disempowerment, disparagement, ignoring, imposition, infantilization, intimidation, invalidation, labelling*).

Mealtimes

See also *Assisting, Eating, Finger-food*

Mealtimes are an opportunity for shared activity, connection and relaxing together.

You can begin your mealtime with the discussion of what you plan to eat. This can stimulate the desire to eat. Sometimes people with dementia may forget to eat or do not have the sensation of hunger that activates the desire to eat. So utilize all the senses to stimulate appetite: the smell of food cooking, the sight of food being prepared and handling fresh food from fridge to worktop can all stimulate appetite and interest in the meal.

Engage the person you care for in food preparation by thinking ahead to the jobs they can do to participate. Knives are sometimes seen as too much of a risk for people with dementia to handle. However, I have never seen a person with dementia cut themselves using a knife nor hurt anyone else while using a knife preparing food.

During the meal, sit opposite each other if you can so that the person with dementia can watch you eat. If they have problems initiating eating or knowing what the food is, you can model eating behaviour and they will usually be able to commence and follow your lead.

Some believe that music during a meal can provide an atmosphere that is conducive to eating. I have only found it to be a distraction when the person needs all their concentration ability to perform the act of handling and eating food. Do not overload the mealtime with lots of conversation. Keep it simple. However, if the act of eating is not working well, you may find that distracting the person with interesting conversation and helping them eat is sufficient for them to obtain the nourishment from the meal.

If sitting for a meal is not possible for whatever reason, you may find the person with dementia benefits from a *finger-food* approach so they can graze throughout the day rather than try to eat three meals a day.

The main priority with a meal is nourishment. A close second is dignity and social engagement. You may find that what is important about the meal shifts as the person's abilities and needs change. One day nourishment will be uppermost; another day you may give more importance to the social enjoyment of the occasion. Be flexible.

As disability increases you will need to adapt your assistance to the level of help required. Assisting with eating is an art. You may find you are helping the person to eat by placing the food in their mouth if they cannot recognize or use utensils or the food itself.

Use your judgement about the pace of assistance, the amount of food and whether to use a fork or spoon. You may also need to monitor for swallowing so that any problems swallowing are picked up early and the consistency of food can be adjusted. Watch for facial expression and level of interest to show you when to stop trying. Come back later. Again, grazing may prove to be a better option than a full meal.

Medication

See also *Antipsychotic medication, Antidepressant medication, Anti-anxiety medication*

Memory problems may make it difficult for the person to remember to take medication or to remember that they have taken it already today. As a caregiver, you will probably need to be responsible for daily medication administration. Check with the GP and your pharmacy/drugstore for ways to reliably administer medication.

Memory

See *Short-term memory, Long-term memory, Forgetting*

Mirroring

Mirroring is a technique that can help a person with dementia to perform actions that they would not be able to do on their own. The presence of another person who is doing the action is often enough to stimulate the person with dementia to do the action. For example, knitting may have been an old well-learned skill but because the person can no longer initiate behaviour they do not knit when on their own. However, if a person knits in the room with them, they may pick up knitting needles and wool and knit as they always have done.

This relies on mirror neurons in the brain that respond to actions that a person sees others do. These neurons also respond to emotions. This is why seeing a person cry makes us sad. It is the basis for empathy and compassion. It can help with eating, dressing, washing, and any activity that the person knows how to do but has lost the starter motor for.

Mirrors

Mirrors can stimulate angry responses. If the person with dementia looks in the mirror they may fail to recognize themselves. They may mistake themselves for a relative from an earlier time in life, particularly if they now look like their parent. Or they may become angry at a stranger they believe is now in their house.

> An elderly gentleman with dementia who was a boxer in his youth walks into a lift with a full-length mirror on the rear wall. On entering the lift he shapes up to the figure in the mirror and begins to challenge him to fight. It takes considerable effort on behalf of the caregiver to prevent him from hitting out at the figure in the mirror, who he sees being equally ready for a fight.

Often the simplest solution is to cover mirrors to prevent them from being a source of agitation or aggression. Alternatively, you may wish to remove the mirrors altogether.

Mistakes

Mistakes are inevitable when a person has dementia because the brain does not support the person to do what they have previously known how to do successfully. One of the most common mistakes is forgetting. Others include spilling liquids, misplacing objects and getting actions out of order.

In dementia care, mistakes are only mistakes in the eye of the beholder. It is important that you as a caregiver do not give too much importance to mistakes. A person with dementia makes mistakes all day, but from their perspective they are trying to live life well and doing what they have always known how to do. These are efforts to live.

If you don't regard these moments as mistakes but simply as how the person is right now, these moments can lose the negative quality for them and for you. Unless there is a safety issue, let it go. What is the point of reminding the person that they have forgotten again? What is the point of pointing out each time they get something wrong or put the knives in the fridge or the milk in the pantry?

People with dementia can still learn, so there may be some value in reinforcing where things go. However, you must weigh the value of this against the cost to their self-esteem and to your relationship. Too much criticism will corrode trust and cause the person to withdraw and shut down. This may only add excess disability to an already difficult situation.

Misunderstood, being

Being misunderstood can create a strong negative reaction of withdrawal, irritation or anger. It may be that you become angry at their mistake and tell them so. They feel misunderstood because it was not their intention to make a mistake. Being blamed for it feels unfair.

Criticism of the person with dementia for mistakes only damages their self-esteem and creates distance. It won't improve their performance.

It may make it more difficult for a person with dementia to make themselves understood if they already have word-finding problems or mix up sentences. This can be very frustrating for them. Listen for the meaning, the tone, the mood of what they are saying. I have had numerous conversations with people who have had severe expressive problems, in which they have been successful because both of us have 'got the gist' of what we meant. Sometimes the 'gist' is all you need.

Mobility, loss of

Brain changes in dementia affect all areas of brain function, including those responsible for movement. Trips, slips, stumbles, falls and difficulties gripping and manipulating objects are more common with dementia. You can help by ensuring that footwear is appropriate and that flooring surfaces are clear of hazards such as black mats (which can look like a hole) and folds in loose carpet. Changes from one surface to another can cause problems. Small objects low down can also be a cause of stumbling.

Mocking

Mockery is to make fun of someone in a demeaning way. Mockery is one of the negative behaviours that can create an environment that is malignant, harmful and hurtful for the person with dementia. It is harmful for anyone to be treated in this way. It causes people to withdraw and lose confidence. If you can, as a caregiver, keep it away from the person you care for.

Mother

See 'Attachment', 'Attachment, caregiving and dementia' and 'Advice giving' in Part I, and *Art* in Part II

Motivation for behaviour

See also 'Needs', Part I: Comfort, Occupation, Attachment, Identity and Inclusion

Ask yourself regularly what is the motivation for the person's behaviour. Look for the reason. There will always be one. It's a matter of searching to find it.

LIVING WITH A PERSON WITH DEMENTIA

What is the person wanting to achieve? What need is the person attempting to satisfy? Tom Kitwood (1997) identified five fundamental needs that motivate people with dementia: comfort, occupation, attachment, identity and inclusion. Each of these needs is discussed in detail in 'Needs', Part I.

Music

Music is a vital source of joy, relaxation and motivation. It is associated with memories of times we heard this or that song. This will date me: I was driving an ancient van each day of a holiday job during the Australian summer of 1979 and will always associate the songs *Roxanne* and *Sultans of Swing* with the long hot days of that youthful summer. I have glimpses of houses I worked at and people I worked for. I remember the feel of the van, I can see its dull grey paint job, how I was dressed, and the kind elderly widow I stayed with that summer. I only have to hear *Sultans of Swing* on the radio now to be plunged into memories and the feel of that summer.

You have preferences for styles of music and songs that make you feel calm, comfortable, excited, joyful, moved to tears. Perhaps it is Elvis, or Mozart or Brahms, or Dire Straits. Whatever the music, the person with dementia will also be moved to remember, to feel. Music can be a wonderful source of reminiscence. It can also be a stimulus to dance, to move, perhaps to dance with you. Be ready to go with it and join in.

Music can be therapeutic. It can help you heal, remember and change mood. It can move you to get out of your chair and dig the garden. Utilize the kind of music the person with dementia likes and wants to listen to or benefits from as a way to change mood. Experiment. You may find you have to try various types of music and it may be that their current preference is unexpected. It may be that they like rap or Indie-rock or hip-hop. As my son-in-law says, 'Whatever floats your boat.'

With platforms like Spotify, you can develop playlists to use for different circumstances. A calm list for times of stress. An upbeat one for times you want to generate action and motivation. A quiet list for moments of rest. If you can't master the mysteries of playlists, you may need to ask a 13-year-old to help you!

Nagging

Avoid nagging. If you don't get a response to the first couple of attempts to get the person with dementia to do something, such as take a shower/bath, you may be better off finding another way to achieve your goal, rather than just repeatedly asking them. Step back from it and rethink your approach.

Nagging just annoys the other person and is counter-productive. It builds resistance and the person may become less and less cooperative. Utilize some of the approaches described in Part I to draw the person towards the desired goal (having a shower/bath) or away from what they are currently doing (watching TV). Use reward to entice. Or come back later and try again. Be patient. For instance, wait until they are preparing for bed and use the opportunity of them being in the bathroom to introduce the idea of a shower/bath.

Nakedness

You may not be comfortable with nakedness – yours or the person you care for. However, it may become more frequent that the person with dementia wants to walk around the house naked or wants to strip off clothing at inopportune times. This can happen because they are unaware of their nakedness, or it may be that they feel uncomfortable in clothes in that moment.

Around the house may not be such a problem if it's just the two of you. However, socially this can be a problem. Use distraction, and engage in other tasks or activities. If the temperature is too high and being hot is the reason for stripping off, adjust the temperature.

If stripping happens in public, keep calm and maintain the person's dignity as much as possible. The calmer you are the better they will cooperate with you. What is the worst that can happen? Other people may see the person naked. Okay, not ideal, but it is not life or death. Keep a perspective about it and take the calm actions you need to in order to maintain dignity and privacy. If others see you take charge, they will be calm and not over-react to it.

Names

See also 'Identity', Part I

Your name is important to you. It carries your identity and activates a sense of self and of being recognized by others, positioned in a social place relative to others. It is the same for the person with dementia. Their name is an important way to affirm their identity. This is one of the five fundamental needs that motivate us and shape our sense of being loved and valued. Avoid nicknames unless that is how they are generally known and unless you have pet names for each other.

Avoid terms of endearment such as darling, love, pet, sweetheart, unless these are names you usually use with each other. It is appropriate to use such names between equals such as spouses, but it is not okay for a much younger caregiver to use with an elder. It has a patronizing and infantilizing tone to it.

Using the person's name usually helps them to remember who they are.

Needs

See 'Needs', Part I

Negotiation

There will be many moments in a caregiver's day when the ability to negotiate is a valuable asset. Negotiation is engaging in a process to reach agreement. This is preferable to you imposing your will on the person with dementia. *Imposition* is often relatively easy to do as you may have the better verbal skills and be able to tell them or convince them they should do what you want. However, this creates an imbalanced and unequal relationship if it is used all the time. There may well be times when this is a last resort but should not be your 'go to'.

Negotiation requires you to adopt an approach as an equal with the person with dementia. Caregiving is a partnership of equals in which your role is to guide and assist, not impose. It often means finding another solution to the shared problem. For instance, if *hygiene* is the issue (and it often is), then the question is how to achieve it. If the person with dementia does not want to get undressed for a shower it is important that you find out what is behind this resistance. There is always a reason. Find out the reason and you are half-way home. To find out the reason from someone who cannot tell you with words means you will need to ask good questions.

Perhaps they do not know the reason for their own resistance to the shower/bath. It may be that the bathroom is cold. If this is the case, warm up the bathroom well before the time it is to be used. If the person does not like the process of undressing as it is effortful and confusing, perhaps you can use music to distract and move the person into a positive mood, or assist them to undress. Or if privacy is an issue, you can give them privacy as they require, checking every so often to see they are safe and engaging in the shower/bath.

Make it simple for them to do what you want to have happen. Break down the task into small steps so they are not having to mentally grasp a complex task that feels overwhelming and anxiety-provoking.

Make it more attractive to do it than not do it. As the old saying goes, 'You get more flies with honey than vinegar.' Perhaps use the idea that they may smell nice and look really attractive for the shopping trip if they have a shower/bath. This may be better than telling them they will smell bad and people will not want to be near them if they don't have a shower/bath.

This means taking some time to reach an agreement. Give yourself enough time to achieve this so you are not trying to do personal hygiene at the last minute before a trip to the shops. Plan ahead so you are not under pressure and you don't put the person with dementia under pressure.

Negotiate and think ahead. Don't impose.

Noise

See also *Agitation*

Noise agitates people. If you notice the person with dementia has become agitated, think about noise as a possible cause. It may be the noise of grandchildren, which can be high-pitched and loud. Or it may be shopping centre noise, which is like a wall of sound from which there is no escaping. This type of noise is also perceived as difficult to make sense of. If we can make sense of a sound, we can tolerate it better, but if it seems pointless, we can be less tolerant of it.

Think ahead about the likely amount of sound the situation will involve. This is also important if the person has hearing difficulties. If they are hard-of-hearing, invite them to sit with their back to a wall, and avoid cafes with hard floors. It can be trial and error to work out which places are better for you both.

Conversation in a room with family can become overwhelming for people with dementia. It may be better to offer a walk in the garden to break up time in a loud family gathering.

Non-verbal communication

People with dementia experience language changes. It is a hallmark of dementia. Non-verbal communication takes on more importance as a way of communicating meaning.

Non-verbal communication consists of body language and prosodic elements of language. Body language is your facial expression, posture, gesture, eye movement and body movement.

Prosody is the sound, rhythm, tone, stress and pitch of speech. In other words, it is how you say it. It matters in communication between two people who do not have dementia, so it matters even more when dementia is a factor.

People with dementia become adept at picking up on non-verbal communication. The brain wants to pick up meaning, so it uses whatever channels it has available and builds skill in these channels. Try to remember as a caregiver that you can influence the outcome of your interactions by managing your own communication. Try to face the person so your facial expressions and tone of voice can be clearly understood. This is not always possible, so be clear with tone in your voice. If you know from experience that the person you care for is likely to pick up on ambiguity and be easily confused about what you mean, be clear, smile and use a relaxed tone.

Objectification

Objectification refers to treating a person as if they were an object, the act of dehumanizing a person. It also refers to degrading them, as if they have no feelings or perspective of their own. In the media, this term is often used in relation to objectification of women as sex objects.

In dementia care, objectification can take the form of talking across someone, moving them without consulting them first, referring to them as a bed-blocker or a full-feed or a shower. The person is reduced in your speech to being a task or an impediment. This is disempowering and demeaning. It results in the person disappearing from your view. You will no longer see the person for who they are.

Work against this tendency. Always consult, check with the person before you invite or assist them to move. Use their name. Include them in decisions. Continue to speak warmly and take the time to ask their opinion or preference.

Obsessions

An obsession is a thought, impulse or image that continually intrudes or occupies a person, and that is persistent. In dementia, they are not necessarily a sign of obsessive compulsive disorder but of a tendency to focus on certain thoughts, impulses or images excessively, which preoccupy the person to the extent that they interfere with the person's ability to carry out daily functions. In other words, they take up time and prevent the person from being available to shift from one activity to another.

An example of such an obsession includes parents, particularly mothers, and the need to get home to mother. Other examples are gathering objects, and fear of particular people.

As a caregiver, you can reassure, distract and engage the person in activities that are enjoyable and satisfy the needs that drive such obsessions. Identify the need that drives it and you will be half-way home.

Occupation

This is one of the five fundamental needs identified by Tom Kitwood (1997). It is the need to be effective in the world, to be able to do stuff like they used to, without being corrected. This need is vital to give expression to a sense of agency, to feel like one's old self and to be productive.

As a caregiver, look for opportunities to engage and include the person in productive activity. Perfect or faultless performance is not the goal. The goal is a sense of well-being. Just doing it without judgement or critique is the means to achieving this sense of well-being. For example, invite the person to help rake the leaves by offering them a rake to hold. You model the raking action and involve them in it. You go about the job and see that they commence raking. Whether it leaves a clean lawn is not the point. But standing back at the end and saying, 'Thanks, that's great. You've been a great help' – that's the point.

Outbursts

Emotional outbursts may happen from time to time. They usually indicate that the person is overwhelmed and unable to contain the amount of feeling they have in them at that time. Perhaps it has been building, and if they are naturally a person who holds feelings in, they may have reached their threshold. Because of cognitive impairment they may not be able to make sense of the experience of emotion in their body or know what do with it. Old defensive habits of projection or externalizing may lead them to explode at others or just explode without a target, or explode at themselves.

Such outbursts require a careful response. Initially, make sure the person is safe and not about to hurt themselves or others, or use objects to throw. Then offer quiet understanding and reassurance. Avoid telling the person off at all costs. Do not criticize them for the outburst. It is appropriate at times to state a limit, such as: 'Please don't shout at me.' This is not focused on the person, but on the behaviour.

Address the issue by waiting for a clue as to what it is about. When you have an idea of the cause, address it simply. It may not be necessary or wise to put it into words (for example, 'You are angry about not being able to get dressed'). Rather than put this difficulty into words that confront the person with their inability, offer a solution such as 'I can hold it for you if you like', 'Try this...' or 'Perhaps do one thing at a time. Here's your shirt.'

Avoid remonstrating with the person as you hear angry parents doing with upset children in a supermarket. They are not children and do not need to be 'told off' or corrected. They need understanding, reasonable limits, patient acceptance and a way forward.

Outpacing

Going too fast for a person with dementia is known as outpacing. This term was coined by Tom Kitwood (1997) to describe the habit of carers to work or assist at a pace that is uncomfortable for people living with dementia.

Working too fast, talking too fast or in too complicated a manner, or asking one question after another without waiting for a response can promote a feeling of failure, inability and inadequacy. Outpacing can be subtle. It is a look of frustration or exasperation when a person with dementia is slower than you would like. Or it could be an overt comment: 'Come on, David. I haven't got all day.' It makes people very uncomfortable and causes them to hurry in order to satisfy you or avoid you becoming angry with them.

Assist at a pace that is driven by the person with dementia and in an atmosphere of warmth and acceptance. This will generate well-being and willingness to make attempts, which can result in more frequent use of existing skills. If the person is accepted as they are and for what they can do, they are more likely to be willing to try to do things and maintain skills and abilities.

Overeating

See also *Eating, Mealtimes*

Overeating can occur when the appetite regulation mechanism in the brain doesn't work as it should. This may be due to a frontal lobe problem and is common in fronto-temporal dementia. We usually are able to sense 'fullness' which signals us to stop eating.

However, this requires self-monitoring and self-awareness and this may not be working. Problems with overeating include excessive weight gain, diabetes and inactivity.

There are a number of things you can do. Provide several small meals during the day so appetite is satisfied. Place small amounts of food out so the person can have access to food regularly in small amounts. Include regular exercise in daily routines and perhaps do this away from food. Provide water so the person can drink but monitor for excessive water consumption, as this can cause problems with electrolyte balance and kidney function. Engage with your GP to monitor progress. It may be necessary to limit the amount of food the person has access to by modifying the types of food (low calorie) and locking food away. I know of a wife who had to put a lock on the fridge and pantry to prevent her husband with dementia eating to excess. This frustrated him and he searched for food throughout the house. I suggest it may be better to use a range of approaches before you go to the locksmith.

Pain

Pain is a problem in dementia as it is frequently under-diagnosed. This is often due to stigma. There is a tendency among medical professionals to interpret signs of pain as being due to dementia and so minimize it or treat it with psychotropic medication rather than pain relief. It is also due to failure of health professionals to take pain seriously in people who have dementia and to misattribute pain signals to behavioural disturbance. If behaviour changes, a key question is always: 'Is there pain for any reason, that may be causing this behaviour?'

People with dementia often have difficulty communicating pain. They may have difficulty finding the words to describe it, and so are dependent on the people around them to pick it up and act on the signals. The most common pain signals are facial expressions, postural and movement changes and behaviour change.

There is a simple FACES pain assessment tool which can be useful for a home caregiver as it is easy to use and you can note the progress of pain signs for visiting health professionals so they have a sense of how the pain is changing over time. It uses facial expressions to show smiles and grimaces that indicate progressively worse pain. You can find copies with an internet search for 'FACES pain scale'.

Toothache can be a cause of behavioural difficulties. Ensure that the person you care for has an annual dental check.

Inactivity can also result in pain, particularly if the person is accustomed to being active and is forced to lie in bed for days at a time due to illness. This can result in back pain or muscle wasting, with weakness and stiffness. You can manage this by ensuring that the person's limbs are moved regularly and by consulting a physiotherapist for a treatment plan.

Use pain relief medication as prescribed and in a timely way, particularly if you are given medication to use 'as needed'. Use it so that pain does not 'break through' and cause distress.

Palliative care

Palliative care is commonly understood as something that occurs at the end of life. However, this is not true.

Palliative care is the prevention and treatment of symptoms and side-effects of life-threatening disease. In these terms, dementia is a condition that qualifies as needing a palliative approach. The focus of palliative care for dementia is to improve and sustain quality of life by preventing and treating the symptoms of dementia. What you do as a caregiver is to adopt a palliative approach. This may be doing all the good things described in this book in an effort to decrease problems and support well-being over the course of the dementia.

End-of-life care is provided in the last few weeks or months of life when physical comfort and management of psychological distress become the primary foci of efforts by specially trained nurses. See *End of life*.

Parents

Early *attachment* figures are frequently the focus for people with dementia as memory for current events and current attachments is more difficult to sustain and past events and people become more available in long-term memory.

The relationships of those early years preoccupy the person with

LIVING WITH A PERSON WITH DEMENTIA

dementia. Getting home in time or before dark, getting things right, being a good girl/boy, pleasing a parent, gaining approval, avoiding a punishing parent or simply being with a parent become preoccupations. Whatever the preoccupations of childhood were, they seem to return and become the emotional focus in the present.

Early attachment relationships with parents set the emotional tone and the template for how the person understands they should feel in order to belong in their family. This has been explored in detail in Part I. In order to belong, to be loved and safe, babies and children work out whether they should be quiet, be invisible, hold their emotions away from mum or dad, not cry, be a good boy/girl, not be a 'nuisance' to their parents, be perfect/faultless, do as mum or dad tells them. Parents set the emotional tone and 'rules' for surviving in the family. In dementia, the person you care for may return to a preoccupation with this early time in their lives when parental figures were dominant and doing what parents wanted was the priority.

As a caregiver, how do you respond? Initially, get a sense of what the preoccupation is, who the person thinks you are and gain a sense of what they are wanting from you. It may be that you have been associated with and are now mistaken for a past figure such as a parent – you may be perceived to be their mother or father.

Your task is to be in tune with the person you are caring for. That means being alert to their emotions, their perceptions and what they want. There are some key questions to ask yourself:

- What are they feeling? Angry/frustrated, anxious/afraid, sad/grieving?

- What are they perceiving, sensing and understanding of their situation? Are they away from home, are they lost, are they alone and feeling frightened, confused about where they are? How old do they see themselves in this scenario?

- What do they want? To go home, to go home to a parent, to avoid punishment, to seek comfort, to find a lost object, to do something important.

If physical safety is at stake, you must act to protect the person if they seem intent on putting themselves at risk but cannot see this, for example getting to the other side of a busy road through traffic.

Clarity of communication is important here as the person is likely to be in an upset state and needs you to help them work their way back to a calm state. If the person has perceived you as someone else (in other words, has lost connection with you and is in another reality just now), adopt the stance of a neutral bystander who is interested in what is happening.

Ask questions that tease out the person's perception and desires: When do you have to be home? Who will be at home waiting for you? Will they be pleased to see you? What will you do when you get home? How does it feel to go home? Do you like being home? You seem worried; is everything going to be okay when you get home? What is your dad like? What is your mum like?

Your job is to validate their perspective by treating it as real for them. Do not challenge it. Avoid 'why' questions. These are confusing as they ask for a reason, and the person is likely to become irritated by such questions and this could jeopardize their rapport with you. Validation is crucial for the sense of being understood. If the person feels understood, they will be calmer. This will be addressed in more detail in *Validation*.

Passivity

Passivity can be caused by dysfunction in the frontal lobes of the brain. This is the region of the brain that helps initiate activity – the starter motor. If this does not kick a person into action they may sit in one place as if waiting for something to happen. In some ways, this is true. If someone/something does not stimulate the person with dementia into action, they may sit there all day. It can look a lot like *apathy*, as if the person does not care. However, this is not a mood problem. It is a neurological problem.

As a caregiver, your role is to notice it and be the starter motor for the person. Ask a question, give an instruction or make a comment to nudge them into action. For instance: 'What time is it? Is it lunch time yet?', 'It's time for our walk after lunch. Change those shoes and we'll get going' or 'I notice the weeds are growing. Help me with the garden.' You will soon work out how much nudging you need to do to get action.

One of the other reasons for passivity is that it is the person's usual personality, which should not be much of a surprise to you and perhaps not much change from the person's usual behaviour.

Finally, passivity may be caused by loss of confidence due to making frequent mistakes or having to rely on others for help. If this is the reason, it may be important to review your approach to ensure that you are not contributing to the loss of confidence and to protect them from the negativity of others. Also provide as many opportunities for the person to gain confidence by having success as independently as possible.

Pauses in conversation

Some of us feel uncomfortable with silence in conversations, to the point we become anxious if the conversation dries up. Words can dry up for some people whether you have dementia or not. If you can be peaceful with a few pauses in the flow of talking, the person with dementia may feel calmer with not having anything to say from time to time. The temptation for some is to fill the silence with words. Avoid this if you can and let the conversation have its natural rhythm. You are not responsible for keeping the flow of words going. If you notice the person with dementia is becoming agitated with the silences, you may need to scaffold the conversation with some prompts that get it going again. With some practice, you can become adept at finding questions or prompts that maintain the flow.

Perception

Your experience of the world outside your brain begins with the channels of sensations that provide you with the raw information: eyes, nose, ears, tongue, skin and inner ear (vision, smell, hearing, taste, touch, balance). It is now recognized that there are several other channels of sensation. These signals provide the raw data for perception.

Your brain is a mechanism for making sense of the signals your senses pick up. It perceives or understands the world through the senses. Your eyes see light and your brain identifies objects and understands how to use them and what they mean to you. You see a locket on a dresser. You perceive that it is your wife's/husband's mother's locket. It has significance for the family as a treasured heirloom. Your ability to perceive the meaning of the object is important because now you can treat it with the respect and value it deserves. You place it carefully in a jewellery box for safekeeping.

However, if your brain is no longer able to process the sensory information reliably, you may not understand the significance of the object. You may find it attractive and put it in your pocket without another thought. It goes through the wash and is found sometime later. The photo inside is ruined. You were unable to perceive or understand the significance of the object. There is no point blaming you as there was no intention to ruin the photo. It was a consequence of a problem with perceiving the significance of it.

Perception problems abound as dementia progresses. As a caregiver, you will come across many instances during a normal day when the person you care for has difficulty perceiving the world around them. It may be recognizing the shirt they are attempting to put on but not recognizing it as a shirt and so placing it over their foot as if it was a trouser leg. It can look comical but it is best to approach it in a low-key way: 'How about you put these on first (handing the person the trousers)?' Or it may be the food they are eating that they do not identify as food.

False perceptions can also occur. These are known as *hallucinations*. Seeing things that are not there and treating them as real. Hearing things that are not there. Sensing insects crawling under your skin, or tastes when there is nothing there. These can be very disturbing and require sensitive response from you to provide reassurance and comfort. Do not attempt to persuade the person that the experiences are not real. Instead, assure them they are safe and that you cannot see or hear what they are seeing. If you think the person may be open to it, ask them what they are seeing. Sometimes the person with dementia may be resistant to describing the experience or treating it as not real. Take their lead and follow what they want. Reassure and provide comfort if they are distressed.

It may be that the person with dementia is not distressed, but is comforted by the presence of the hallucination. A widow living on her own was referred to the Aged Person's Mental Health Team for assessment and treatment of her hallucinations. She was seeing small people on the curtain rail every evening. They appeared reliably and sat there talking to her every evening. She would not reveal what they spoke about but she told the nurse that she looked forward to them coming and always slept well. They watched TV with her and reappeared the next evening.

She had found a natural way to overcome her loneliness and isolation. Should she have been prescribed medication? The hallucinations were not causing distress. They alleviated it. So, when you are faced with a person with dementia experiencing hallucinations, first determine if they cause distress. If not, probably just monitor the situation for any changes as time passes. Identify the fundamental need the hallucinations satisfy and perhaps consider providing another way to satisfy that need. For instance, the widow may have benefitted from connection to local groups or a regular visiting service or support group.

Personality

Much has been written about personality that is readily available elsewhere. This section will simply acknowledge that personality does affect the way dementia progresses in a person. People who have high neuroticism (are prone to anxiety and worry) do tend to find dementia more distressing and overwhelming. They need reassurance and comfort to get through the day and may be clingy and need your presence to feel calm.

Extroverted people tend to become more socially engaged but have difficulty following through the interactions with others successfully due to word-finding problems. The desire for contact and interaction may be still there but the wherewithal may not be. You may need to scaffold the experience to provide opportunities for success.

Personality can change significantly in dementia. A person who is passive can become socially active. A bossy person can become quiet and passive. Some conditions cause rapid and significant personality change. These include Lewy body disease and other frontal lobe dementias. Some people will become suspicious or depressive in their outlook.

Personality changes can be distressing for family members. There may be periods of rapid change and then stability or it may be progressive and continuous. The person is still there and you will see glimpses of their former self as it were; however, it may be difficult to find consistency in how they act now compared to pre-dementia. Be patient and talk about it with trusted friends or family. Take breaks for yourself. If this is difficult due to lack of support it may be time to consider linking with some outside organizations such as the Alzheimer's Association or other carers' support groups in your local area.

Person-centred care

This is an approach to caregiving that has developed over the past 40 years and become regarded as the gold standard for dementia care. It takes many forms but has at the core a focus on the value, individuality, perspective and social needs of the person being cared for. These four dimensions of the person-centred approach were identified by Professor Dawn Brooker (2015) and are known as the VIPS approach to person-centred care.

- *Value:* The person is valuable no matter how impaired and disabled they become. They have an intrinsic worth as a human being that cannot be taken away by loss of memory, or ability to pay taxes or contribute to society financially or intellectually.

- *Individuality:* The person is unique and has likes/dislikes, priorities and needs, characteristics that are unique to them. They have a history, a life story that makes them who they have become. It may be that they have served in a war, parented children or contributed to development of ideas. They have a unique personality that makes them the particular person they are.

- *Perspective:* The person has a perspective, or point of view, that is often lost under the weight of assumptions and the priorities of others who think they know best what a person with dementia wants or should have or do. Their point of view can be easily lost with word-finding and memory problems that make expression of this perspective difficult or impossible. It is often up to us to preserve the perspective and repeatedly scaffold space for it to be heard.

- *Social needs:* The person has a vital and core need to be social for their sense of self. We are made for relationship. It is in relationship with others from the womb that we become the unique person we are. Person-centred care supports the social capacities and opportunities the person needs to continue flourishing as a social being.

Personhood

No matter how impaired by dementia a person may be and how changed they are by it, they retain their personhood. This is the dignity and value they have as a human person. It does not diminish with the changes to the person's abilities.

Caregivers face the challenge of looking beyond the changes and behaviour or the person to the person themselves. Thomas, Ibrahim and Joan all remain Thomas, Ibrahim and Joan. Their essence does not disappear. But they do change.

We all develop through life. You are not the same as you were at age 20 years. Yet you are the same person. Giving birth, raising children, living life – all these shape and change you so that you mature and develop as a person. Life events can change us for good or for ill. Some people become depressed by life or anxious and overwhelmed. Some become embittered and negative; others confident and grateful. So, too, dementia changes a person. But it is change due to a disease process rather than the range of normal life events. Even in the face of this disease process your personhood, your dignity as a human person, is not diminished.

Personhood is a quality that exists in us and is not extinguished by life, illness or disability. Tom Kitwood (1997) talked of personhood as a standing or status that we accord others by being in a relationship with them. It requires a recognition of that person, a respect for them and engagement in a relationship of trust. He wrote of bestowing it on others. The idea of recognition is important here. It is there in the other person and is recognized by us. We have to be able to see it. As a caregiver, the challenge is to not let the daily care tasks get in the way of recognizing the personhood, dignity and respect due the other person, regardless of what they have done or not done.

Photographs

Memory changes mean that photographs become a useful prompt for reminiscence. Perhaps consider having photos around the house and developing a life-story book that can be a daily or at least regular means of activating memory and connection for the person with their own personal life story. It can be valuable to place a simple statement beside each photo with who is in it and when it was taken or how it fits into the person's life. Engage family members in developing this life story.

If you are concerned that the originals of precious photos may be damaged if handled regularly, make copies and install these in photo frames. Perhaps keep the originals elsewhere. Old photos will be valuable prompts as they will stimulate long-term memories.

When showing photos to someone with dementia, give them the names of each person or at least provide some names so it prompts memory. Avoid asking them, 'Who is that?' It's a pointless test and only creates a probable failure. Better to provide the name and stimulate the association.

Physical environment

Much has been written about how residential settings such as nursing homes should be designed for people living with dementia. However, if you are caregiving at home, there are also some elements to bear in mind.

Way-finding is an ability we take for granted. This becomes difficult in dementia, so provide physical or pictorial cues to help the person find where they need to go in the house. It may be as simple as a written sign on the toilet door. Or if they can no longer read, it may be a graphic of a toilet seat, or perhaps an old-style toilet.

Signs on drawers and cupboards can be useful prompts to help locate where to find the knives and forks for setting the table or when emptying the dishwasher. It may also be useful to consider replacing the cupboard fronts with clear Perspex fronts so the person can see what goes where.

Fit night-lights throughout the house so the person can find

LIVING WITH A PERSON WITH DEMENTIA

their way at night. Light receptivity may change in dementia so that the person may need more light by which to read or sit, but they may find glare difficult to deal with. Modify the settings as necessary to ensure that the person can function comfortably.

Ensure that the house is secure, and that windows and doors can be locked and not opened without a key. This is important to prevent the person leaving the house unaccompanied at night in particular, but also during the day.

Walking safely throughout the house can be difficult if you have several changes in floor surfaces and levels. Avoid trip hazards by ensuring that flooring is not too slippery and that objects are not left where they can be tripped over. Also check that shoes are suitable for the person so they can walk safely, providing enough grip but not too much. Steps and stairs can be a problem that requires monitoring.

Fences are an important safety feature. It may be that you need to consider how to ensure that the person cannot get through gates unaccompanied. Be aware that a fence can be a challenge to some people. Scaling it can be seen as a triumph and the frailest person may be able to summon the energy and ingenuity to succeed. You may need to consider having the person wear a personal tracking device. In recent years these have become small and fitted into watches and the like. It may be less restrictive and less risky than locking a gate, resulting in the person trying to scale a fence to achieve their freedom.

Smells of food preparation can be a good source of stimulation for appetite. Most houses are of a scale that kitchen aromas can be smelled anywhere in the house. If this is not the case, you may need to take a dish to where the person is in order to stimulate appetite and get them to come to the dining room.

Temperature can be a cause of agitation if it is too high or too low. Open windows for fresh air and cooling. The person may need to be assisted to dress according to the weather.

Play

Relaxation and pleasurable times are important to create a balance for you both when you are caring for someone with dementia.

There can be wonderful moments of closeness and joyfulness. You cannot make mistakes when you play. Perhaps a life-story book will stimulate some happy memory. Or throw autumn leaves up in the air together. Creating opportunities for playfulness is important for your own and their health.

Positioning

We position each other by how we talk about and to each other. I position myself as an expert or as a student by how I dress, how I speak, how I introduce myself and how I am addressed. Social positioning affects people with dementia to a significant degree.

Listen for the sing-song tone and raised pitch as people speak to those with dementia as if they are children. The actual words also change and become diminutive: 'Hello darling, are you going for a little walk?' This is patronizing and positions the person as a child. Watch for the word 'little'. It diminishes the significance of what the person is doing.

Social positioning can locate the person as someone who knows nothing and never had a career or achievements, is a cipher or a non-human entity. Or it can locate the person as a veteran whose war service is respected and valued, as a professor whose knowledge and expertise may still be evident in her speech and concerns, as a mother whose nurturing ability is still ready to hand, as a sister who has been loyal and loving.

Knowing something about the person can give you a perspective on them that enables you to position them in a way that respects their personhood, their social and professional identity. For example, the farmer who knew seasons and can still sense the changes in the weather and knows the activities he did this time every year for 60 years; the carpenter who runs his hand over wooden furniture as he passes and mumbles, 'Walnut, quarter-sawn. Lovely.'

How do you position the person you care for by the way you speak to them? How can you improve the social positioning you contribute to? Where do you hear others do it to the person you care for?

Positive and Negative Signs Scale (PANSIS)

This is a scale used to measure the frequency and severity of signs of well-being and signs of ill-being, based on those first identified by Tom Kitwood (1997). Each sign is rated on a scale of 1–5. The signs are listed in the Appendix.

Positive person work

Positive person work is a term coined by Tom Kitwood (1997) to describe specific person-centred care actions that enhance the well-being of people living with dementia. They include *validation*, *empowerment*, *recognition* and *inclusion*, each of which is examined in this book.

Post-traumatic stress disorder (PTSD)

People can have PTSD if they have experienced or witnessed life-threatening situations. It used to be known as 'shell-shock' and 'combat fatigue' but can occur to anyone who experiences trauma. This includes war veterans, prisoners of war and survivors of rape/sexual assault, natural disasters, terrorist acts, long-term intimate partner violence. It is increasingly well recognized by health professionals and the general public.

It is estimated by the American Psychiatric Association that one in 11 people will experience PTSD in their lifetime. Women are twice as likely to have PTSD as men. It is more common among US Latinos, African Americans and Native Americans/Inuit than non-US Latino whites (Taylor-Desir, 2022). It can occur at any age.

A diagnosis of PTSD must include the following:

- Symptoms of re-experiencing the traumatic event(s). This includes flashbacks, intrusive thoughts and memories that are so real to the person that they relive the experience.

- Avoidance of reminders of the event(s). People may avoid going to places that remind them of the event, and avoid talking about it.

- Changes in mood and thinking. This includes being unable to remember parts of the experience (going blank), or thinking distorted thoughts about themselves (I'm hopeless, I'm to blame) or others (No one can be trusted).

- Hyperactivation of senses and arousal system that results in anxiety about strangers, excessive fear, angry outbursts or irritability, being watchful, suspicious and easily startled.

In dementia, it may be that past events are confused with current events. Memory can become distorted and past trauma can be re-experienced as current. This can become a problem at night and during personal care activity.

At night, it may be that the person with dementia wakes from sleep confused and disoriented and thinks you are part of the enemy force or that you are trying to restrict them or betray them. This can be dangerous for you and you should attempt to make yourself safe, and calm the person if you can.

If you know that war or past civilian trauma is likely to cause episodes of agitated confusion, you may have to prepare the house so that the person has no access to sharp objects at night and doors are locked so they cannot flee the house while you are asleep. Ensure that the person has no access to guns in the house.

Most of the time you will be able to calm the person and they will return to sleep. However, this can be draining emotionally for you and it may be difficult for you to then go back to sleep. Do not keep these events to yourself. Talk to a friend or a health professional so that someone knows what you are dealing with.

Personal care is the other time that past traumatic events can influence current behaviour. It seems that the close proximity in a private space such as a bathroom, or dressing and undressing, can activate past experience. If sexual assault/rape has been a part of their life, you may have to take this into account by reassuring, avoiding nakedness, ensuring that they have as much control over the situation as possible, going slowly, keeping your voice calm and pleasant and stopping if there are signs of agitation or distress.

The person with dementia may be activated by the presence of a new carer if you are taking respite leave. If you know you are going on respite, ensure that there is sufficient overlap so that the new carer is not a stranger.

Power battles

'Do you want to be right or happy?' I'm not sure where I first heard this piece of marriage counselling advice but it is also appropriate here. Power battles end with one winner and one loser. That loser is the person you care for. Avoid these if you can as they corrode trust and make it difficult to work or live together afterwards. They are usually a conflict of wills in which you each see a situation differently and feel the need to have your way.

About the only reason you may need to win a battle with the person is for physical safety, and even then, there is usually more than one way to achieve this. You do not need to butt heads to make the person safe. Come up with alternatives. Work around it. For instance, if the person wants to wear three jumpers and you think they will overheat on an already warm day, turn the air-conditioning down, so the temperature suits what they have chosen to wear. Or start some exercise that requires them to move about, meaning they need to remove one or more of the jumpers. If you don't have air-conditioning, consider cool drinks and introduce changing clothes to go out shopping or for an activity. Every other situation can be negotiated or let go. Ask yourself if it is really important in the grand scheme of things. Most of the time you will find it is not.

Privacy

Having dementia does not reduce a person's need for privacy. Usually in life, toilet and bathroom (bathing) activity is private. As a principle, privacy should continue to be respected. However, because there may be a need for assistance in these activities, it is important to negotiate or slowly introduce the idea of you being involved for part or all of what is usually a private activity.

It depends what the problem is. For instance, if a person does not clean themselves adequately after the toilet, you may notice a smell to which they are oblivious. How you approach this topic may depend on how well you know the person, how much trust and bond there is between you both. You may have to be assertive and gentle at the same time. And be ready to back off and try again or simply 'rip the band-aid off' and deal with it. It depends on the importance of the problem and your relationship. Or you may call out from the other side of the door, 'Remember to wipe yourself/dry yourself. The job is not finished till the paperwork is done.'

You may see the need before the person does, so initially be patient and suggest you are there to help or remind them of the need for cleanliness or *hygiene*. Then point out a benefit of having some assistance. One of the benefits of assistance is that it alleviates a problem for the person. But you may have to point out that there is a problem so they can see the benefit.

If a person with dementia has experienced traumatic stress in their life you may need to be particularly careful about privacy as breaches of privacy in the past may have caused the trauma. These events can be associated with breaches of trust and with *abuse* or *assault*.

Problem behaviour

This has been addressed under numerous headings throughout this book. You will find helpful information in Part I and in *Absconding, Aggression, Attention-seeking, Challenging behaviour, Distress behaviour, Disturbed behaviour, Excess disability, Motivation for behaviour* and *Causes, behavioural.*

Psychological therapies

There has been significant progress in recent decades in the use of psychological therapies with people who live with dementia. These include cognitive behavioural therapy, and psychodynamic therapies. These are both useful therapies, but some conditions apply.

Cognitive behavioural therapy relies on assisting a person to make changes in the way they think and behave. This requires that the person with dementia has sufficient verbal and memory capacity to participate and to remember the strategies from one session to another. They may be able to do this with support of daily reminders to reinforce the work of each session. You, as caregiver, may be an important participant in these sessions.

Psychodynamic therapy focuses on the ways early life experience affects current living. Psychodynamic therapies have a reputation for being long-term and passive, requiring too much intellectual capacity for people with dementia. However, recently short-term active psychodynamic therapies have been used with people with dementia with good outcomes. Psychodynamic approaches now are active and aimed at helping the person to experience feelings that are avoided and blocked. The patterns of blocking and avoiding are usually life-long and link to early life experience. Emotional engagement in the session effectively bypasses the need for intellectual capacity and relies only on the person's ability to participate in the session. Emotional changes take place outside the limits of memory or intellect.

Psychosis

Psychosis consists of *delusions* and *hallucinations*, decrease in self-care and increased disorganization, and can frequently be part of dementia. The loss of brain cells in dementia interrupts the balance of neurotransmitter levels that usually ensure good brain function, and this can result in psychosis. *Antipsychotic medication* is often used as a means of settling agitation that can accompany delusions and hallucinations.

Punishment

Avoid punishing the person at all costs. It is easy to slip into doing it, either in frustration or in an attempt to correct or eliminate the person's behaviour.

Better to use a carrot than a stick, honey rather than vinegar. A person with dementia has enough to deal with without introducing something unpleasant as a punishment for something they have done. There are ways to avoid behaviour that you do not want.

For instance, if a person is repeatedly urinating during a shower or in the bath, provide an opportunity for them to urinate prior to getting in the shower or bath. Avoid the problem in the first place.

Purpose, sense of

A sense of purpose is important to everyone. People with dementia need a sense of purpose just as you who do not have dementia need it. It helps you get out of bed in the morning and can motivate you to work hard to achieve or put effort into your day.

As a caregiver, you may wonder how you can support such a sense of purpose. It can be as simple as setting a time to get out of bed and planning the day ahead. Plan a day together and perhaps a week with special goals or activities that you can both look forward to. Visit art galleries, a zoo, other places of interest to you both. Get together with others who have dementia and their caregivers. Engage with particular people who are friends and organize a meet-up.

Ask yourself what gets you out of bed in the morning. That is part of your sense of purpose.

Quality of life

What makes for a high-quality life? Well, that depends. After a great deal of research, experts have concluded that quality of life for people with dementia consists of several domains: physical, psychological and social.

There are several questionnaires that are commonly used to measure health-related quality of life. The QUALIDEM is one of them. It measures care relationship, positive affect, negative affect, restless tense behaviour, positive self-image, social relation, social isolation, feeling at home, having something to do. So if you think about the quality of life of the person you care for, their relationship with you is an important element of their quality of life. Other elements include how much positive feeling or pleasure and enjoyment they have, how much negative feeling they have, how much restless tense behaviour they have, how positively they see themselves, how connected they are to others, how isolated they are, how relaxed and comfortable they are and how occupied or bored they are.

Reaching through dementia

This may seem like a strange phrase but it refers to the effort you put in to connect to the person through the dementia. Quite often you will only be able to see the dementia and find it difficult to see or connect with the person. At times like these it is valuable to remind yourself of the person who may have become invisible to you. The person is still there but you have to reach out, through the dementia, to get to the person, and then keep the person in mind. You may need to remember something specific that helps you connect, that helps you to keep the person in mind. It may be as simple as saying to yourself, 'What is she feeling?', in order to remind yourself that she has feelings and a perspective on her experience of dementia. Over time, you may have to put more effort into reaching through the increasing dementia to connect with the person.

Reactions to behaviour

Your reactions are an important element in how the person copes with their experience of dementia. If you show frustration each time they get something wrong or make a mistake, it will usually cause them to try to hide their mistakes or deny them. However, if you accept and respond calmly to mistakes and getting things wrong, the person is likely to be more relaxed themselves. Like you, they are doing their best. They are not trying to forget information or put cutlery in the wrong drawer.

Accept them with their mistakes and odd behaviour and you will find a way forward to more peace than if you complain or resent their changed behaviour.

Reading

Reading may become difficult as the skill to recognize letters, words and sentences is eroded. You may find, however, that they still enjoy opening a newspaper and going through the motions of reading.

Reading to the person may be useful here. If they can no longer read the newspaper, they may enjoy you reading certain items to them. Reading books to them can also be valuable as it can become a shared time of peaceful sitting and sharing a story. As concentration will be reduced it may not last a long time but it can be an enjoyable break from activity. Reread familiar stories or parts of stories that you know they have enjoyed in the past. They may or may not find these still enjoyable but, like most strategies, it is worth a try.

Reality orientation

This is an approach to dementia care that was popular for a time but was quickly shown to be rather harsh and did not consider the personal needs of individuals with dementia. For instance, some people with dementia find that being reminded of the death of their loved one is too confronting and upsetting.

Reality orientation is useful when it is focused on providing a context to the person's day, such as details about the season, date, month, time of day and day of the week. It is a valuable way to orient someone when they cannot do it themselves. 'You are Maria. I am your husband Ibrahim and we live here together. We have lived here for 20 years at 2 Hope Street, Yarragon. We have three children: Rebecca, Jonathan and Amin.' This can be calming and reassuring if the person cannot remember it.

However, if the person becomes upset and rejects that you are her husband/wife, let it go, and listen for who the person thinks you are. You may get another chance to affirm that you have a connection and who you are, but if the delusion they are in is too strong you may not be able to until it settles. You may have to attempt to move the person on to something less stressful and more pleasurable.

It is better to use a combination of validation and reality orientation when appropriate. The goal is to maintain the person in a good emotional state. Use whichever approach works to achieve that.

Recall memory

This is a type of memory that enables us to bring to mind knowledge we have already stored. The other related type of memory is *recognition memory*.

Recognition memory

This type of memory enables us to recognize objects or information as familiar even though we may not have been able to recall them.

Recognizing faces

Faces are recognized in a specific part of your brain. When that area of your brain is affected by dementia it becomes difficult to recognize faces, even of familiar and loved people. It may be that the person with dementia is unable to recognize you as their spouse or child. Combined with memory loss, this is a particularly upsetting experience for relatives who rely on being recognized and greeted as part of family relationships.

Being recognized and addressed by your mother/father is important to us from early in life when as children we first got to know our mother's face and then the faces of others such as our father and other family members. To not be recognized now can be devastating for adult children. If the person has younger onset dementia (aged less than 65 years), they may have teenage children living at home still, and this lack of recognition from a parent can be very painful.

If you know this is likely to happen it can be best to announce yourself with your name and who you are to them: 'Hi Dad, it's Josie, your daughter.'

Recreation

Physical activity and relaxation can be ways to engage in recreation. It is an important part of life and may be a useful way to use up energy to ensure a good night's sleep. Recreation may also be engaging in hobbies which a person with dementia can still continue as long as it is physically safe and can be supported. A balanced life with physical activity and periods of rest is important for people with dementia – and for you as caregiver. Ensure that you keep your balance with the four pillars of a healthy life.

Refusal

Refusing to cooperate with your requests, invitations or directions may occur. You may have to find a way around it by backing off and approaching the subject again a little later or by changing the focus of your approach. Even changing your tone can work. Be strategic and avoid a head-on collision. The loser will be your relationship.

Try to identify what it is about your approach to the person that is causing them to refuse. It may be any element of your communication. Or it may have nothing to do with you and everything to do with the fact that they need to go to the toilet and they are uncomfortable.

Regression

Regression in people with dementia may be caused by stress or trauma. It is usually an effort to be cared for by behaving in a child-like way in situations they feel overwhelmed by. It may be crying, following, clinging, or even urinating/defecating. These are signs of attachment need and should be responded to with that in mind.

It is best responded to calmly and with care and warmth. The person needs connection, acceptance and security and is behaving in a way to get you to look after them, provide care and make them feel secure and safe.

Urinating and defecating may also be indications of *anger*, so be alert to the signals that there may be anger behind this behaviour.

Reinforcement

Reinforcement is the process of increasing the likelihood of a behaviour occurring by using a mechanism known as a reinforcer. A reinforcer may be a person, object, words, an activity, a place or an animal. It must be valuable to the person to be effective. They must want it. You can make anything into a reinforcer by linking

LIVING WITH A PERSON WITH DEMENTIA

it to the desired behaviour. For example, if the desired behaviour (what you want to have happen) is that the person with dementia will have a shower before bed, you must link that behaviour with something they want. So when they have a shower, they get the reinforcer. It may be a special food. However, if you give this food all the time, the reinforcer will have little motivational value. In order to obtain this reward, they will have to do the desired behaviour.

This works if it is consistent.

Relationships

Social connections with other people are essential for well-being and quality of life. They help to define who we are as individuals. Try to maintain your own relationships as much as you can throughout your time as a caregiver. You and the person with dementia need your relationships to keep you connected with others, to support your mood and stimulate your mind.

Relatives

Relationships with relatives provide an opportunity for people with dementia to interact with people who are in their long-term memory. Use this familiarity to your advantage by having relatives visit to stimulate old memories, particularly if they have photos. Explain beforehand about how to present photos. Do not quiz the person about who is in the photos. Rather, show the photo and tell them who is in it. Let them contribute to the stories, but scaffold the experience. Avoid a quiz!

Religion

See *Church, Faith, Spirituality*

Religious practice can be a useful way to sustain the person's sense of themselves. Engaging in well-practised rituals of worship can evoke and nourish their identity.

Reminiscence

This is a core activity in dementia care. Looking back over a long life, remembering is often enjoyable and calming and reinforces memories. Stimulus for reminiscence can be photographs, objects from the past, places the person has lived, people they have known.

See *Photographs, Family, Death, Life Story*.

Repair

Seventy per cent of our interactions with each other are misunderstandings or mistakes and require some form of repair to enable the relationship to go on after the interaction (Tronick & Gold, 2020).

Repair is the mending of the rapport and bond you have with the person living with dementia. Emotional injuries occur in every relationship and they will occur in your relationship with the person you care for.

Repair of relationships is an important part of normal socializing and it becomes super important in dementia care. There are more moments of misunderstanding and mistakes in interactions between you and the person with dementia who you care for. You may not be responsible for them, but it will be up to you to repair the relationship so that you can both proceed to the next thing. Repair can be a simple apology or it can be 'Oh, that's what you meant', or it may be a hug or a touch or eye contact, a smile or laughter at a mistake. Do whatever you need to do to ensure that you can both be together after the interaction that went astray.

Repetitiveness

Repetitive questions or statements can go on for a long time and can be very draining for a caregiver. Even though you have answered the question or responded to the remark you may find that the person keeps repeating it over and over again.

If this occurs, it is worth asking why. It may be that the person is stuck in a loop that has its origins in the neurological changes of dementia. For instance, frontal lobe changes can result in difficulty changing set or focus. Or the cause may be that your response is not quite what the person was needing, so they have an unmet need. Understand the need and you can provide the satisfying response. Then you will likely resolve the repetitiveness.

For instance, it may be that the person wants to know where their husband/wife is, and you are their husband/wife. You can gently say who you are, but that may not be enough. If the request is repeated, you may need to think about what it is about you that they want. It may be something unique, such as a song you sing together, or a place you first met or travelled to, that is most memorable. This may stimulate a sense of being with the person they are wanting. Cast around until you find the key and the angst will resolve.

If the repetitiveness is driven by a neurological loop that is not resolvable by activating specific feelings or memories, it may be that it is best responded to with distraction and attempts to shift the person to a more satisfying activity. If this is not effective you may need to consider a medication response. The general principle is that medication is a last resort after psychosocial approaches have been tried.

Repression

Repression is a psychological defence mechanism whose purpose is to keep unacceptable or painful thoughts, memories, feelings and impulses from conscious awareness. For example, past traumatic events may not be remembered even though it would be reasonable to expect the person to be able to remember. This may include childhood abuse or adult assaults, or wartime experience. The definition of a defence mechanism is that it is beyond awareness. The person will not know that they are repressing memories or feelings from awareness.

In dementia, the effectiveness of this defence mechanism can be reduced. Traumatic, distressing experience can then come to consciousness, causing significant upset and confusion to the person; for example, they may believe they are being assaulted in the present rather than it being a past event. This can be distressing for caregivers who get accused of assaulting the person when they have not done so.

If such events resurface into consciousness, provide reassurance and affirm that they are safe with you. Alert any carers coming into the home that personal care activities may stimulate past trauma and ask them to take extra care with bathing, assisting in the toilet, or dressing the person. Take time, avoid rushing, ask permission, keep stress at a minimum and take steps to ensure that the person feels in control of and aware of the process as much as possible. Announce care before you do it, look for signs of refusal or lack of permission before proceeding. Do not assume it is okay to do something for or to the person without their permission, particularly if it involves removing or adjusting clothing.

Other psychological defence mechanisms may also be less effective and cause resurfacing of unwanted past experience at a feeling and memory level. This can include *denial*, which is a common defence.

Repression can often be associated with physical pain or discomfort in the respiratory and digestive tracts. In other words, unacceptable experience is repressed into these physical areas, causing a range of physical problems that have psychological origin. This may include difficulty breathing when under stress, bowel pain, cramping, constipation, diarrhoea and bloating, all of which can be made more severe when the person is under stress from reminders of the unacceptable emotions or memories. If these occur, seek medical opinion to rule-out physical illness.

Reprimand

Don't do it. It is damaging to self-esteem and rapport. Use one of the many other ways in this book to process your displeasure at the person's behaviour.

Respite

See also *Burnout, Guilt*

You need regular breaks from caregiving so that you can continue as long as you are needed in that role. With dementia, this can be for years. You may be in it for the long haul, in which case you will need to organize some respite or breaks so you can recharge your batteries and return to it refreshed.

Local agencies will usually provide respite services. Plan ahead

LIVING WITH A PERSON WITH DEMENTIA

as they are scarce resources. It is important for your own sense of peace and calm that you have periods of respite booked so you can look forward to them. You need something regular as well as occasional nights out or a meal to catch up with a friend. You may decide that you need a holiday and this can also be organized through your respite provider. You may need to organize for the person you care for to stay in a care home for the period of your absence, which can be challenging for you both to come to grips with. It may be the first time you have been separated in many decades. Guilt can be a problem here. Deal with it and go on holiday anyway.

Routine, daily

Daily routine is helpful in reducing the amount of new information the person with dementia has to cope with each day. If the sequence of events in the day is predictable, the person does not have to think or worry about what is going to happen next. Therefore, they are likely to be more settled.

Routine gives structure to your day. The regularity of predictable activity ensures that people can be carried along by it rather than having to expend mental energy coping with new and unpredictable activity. Structure provides rhythm and ensures that changes from one activity to another are predictable and therefore not stress provoking.

Routine is good. However, boredom can become an issue if there is no variation in activity. So, a mix of routine and novel activity can be useful. You do not want to visit the zoo every day, but once a year may be so novel that it is enjoyable if it is with familiar people. Birthdays are enjoyable because they happen once a year. This is a part of a routine though, so we can make a special occasion part of the regular routine. Give people notice of what is to happen so that they can prepare themselves mentally. That said, if they are prone to becoming anxious before a special trip or event, you may want to leave it to the morning of the activity to tell them about it so they do not have time to ruminate and worry.

Sadness

See Part I, and *Bereavement*.

Safeguarding

See also *Abuse, Assault*

Safeguarding is the protection of vulnerable people by using policies and practices that ensure they are protected from harm or abuse. It focuses on promoting well-being, physical and emotional safety and preventing harm.

As a caregiver, you have legal and moral responsibilities to ensure that you are safeguarding from harm and abuse the person you engage with in a relationship of care. It may be useful for you to explore the information online in your country so you are familiar with local definitions and information.

Scaffolding

We scaffold the person by providing enough structure to the experience for them to be successful without taking over.

Examples of scaffolding include putting out the clothes on the bed in the order you want the person to put them on so that underwear is on top; chunking the amount of information you give a person with dementia so they are not overwhelmed by too much at a time; cutting up food so the person can eat it easily; starting them off on an activity so they know the direction and can proceed without having to try to remember how to start. This is scaffolding.

Scaffolding is an important caregiving skill to develop so you can avoid moments of overwhelm and failure and promote success and confidence. It is knowing how to give just the right amount of support at the right time.

Scolding

Don't do it. Self-esteem needs to be cared for and is fragile at the best of times. Hold your temper and your tongue. Verbally scolding the person can cause them to withdraw or react with aggression. As an alternative, if it is physical safety that is a concern, intervene quickly and gently to distract them or remove the danger or risk, or move the person away from the risk. Most other situations require a less urgent response and it is best to ask yourself, 'Is it really important, in the big scheme of things? Is it more important than our rapport?'

Screaming

Screaming can occur if the person has gone over their threshold for what they can tolerate and feels overwhelmed with pain, hunger, thirst, anxiety, sadness or frustration. They may be surrounded by too much noise in the environment. It may be late in the afternoon and they may be depleted and unable to process the stimulation they have around them. It may mean you missed earlier signs of building tension or frustration and didn't head it off in time. Screaming in this case may be a sign to back-off and reset. It can also be caused by an infection such as a urinary tract infection causing a delirium.

First, identify the cause(s). There may be more than one. Is the reason within the person (pain, anxiety, sadness, infection, hunger, thirst or loneliness) or outside the person (noise, absence of someone to help, mirrors) as in Figure 1.2 (Part I)? Second, address any physical needs. These are often quickly met and can resolve the screaming. If it is pain, providing medication may relieve it. Try to identify the cause of the pain and treat that.

Your presence may also be comforting enough to calm the person. Provide comfort in the form of physical care and in the form of your presence. If the person is lonely, sit with them and touch them (hold hands or place your hand so they can touch you), as much as they are comfortable.

Sedation

Sedation is a common unwanted side-effect of medication. It can also be a desirable effect of medication if you are undergoing a medical procedure.

In dementia care, it is unwanted. Sedation reduces alertness and increases confusion. If drugs are given to improve sleep at night, they can also increase sedation during the day. Sedation can be a side-effect of all types of medication that affect thinking and mood, including *antipsychotics, antidepressants* and *anti-anxiety drugs*. Consult your medical practitioner for help with working out the best medication type, amount and timing.

Don't tolerate sedation as it can have a toxic effect on brain function if allowed to remain for some time.

Self

People with dementia retain a sense of self. This is reflected in their thoughts about what they want and how they see their lives. Their reflections on their own memory problems and having dementia can be a valuable way to find out about their inner world. They maintain their inner world just as you and I do.

Our ability to be in touch with this inner world and their ability to express their reflections diminishes if language is impaired. However, non-verbal signs of their mood, wants, desires and preferences will give you indications of their continuing perspective on the world.

An inner sense of self will be revealed in expressions of well-being or ill-being. Tom Kitwood (1997) identified these and they provide a clear indication of contentment and distress.

Self-esteem

What you think of yourself can fluctuate with how you act and receive feedback from others. If you receive feedback that you are making mistakes, your self-esteem will likely plummet. Alternatively, if you receive positive feedback that is realistic praise for real achievements, your self-esteem will be supported and maintained. It only takes one error for you to focus on the negatives and become consumed by them.

You can help to maintain the self-esteem of the person with dementia by listening carefully and being attentive to what they need to remain in a good emotional state. Provide opportunities for success as this can remind them of themselves and what they feel good doing.

Self-harm

Self-harm in dementia most often appears in the first 12 months after diagnosis as people come to grips with the changes in their lives and confirmation of what they may have feared was the case. It is more common in men than in women and more common in people who are separated, divorced or widowed than among married people with a recent diagnosis of dementia.

Social support after diagnosis is crucial to helping the person come to terms with the changes in their lives and the trajectory they are now on. Males tend to cope worse with illness than females and this is reflected in the data about dementia. However, regardless of gender, both men and women need support during the early period after diagnosis.

Sex

Sex is great. Well, most of the time. Okay, occasionally. Rarely? Sex is different for each person, and average figures for frequency of sexual activity such as intercourse are nearly always misleading. Many very happy older couples have not had sexual intercourse for years and are content with their intimate lives together. Others find as they age that sex remains an important part of their lives.

With dementia, sexual activity may change to become more or less frequent. If it is important to the person with dementia, it can become a problem for you as a caregiver if you do not want to participate either as frequently or in the same way. It may be that having sex together gives you an opportunity to be a partner for a few moments, having spent the day being a caregiver. Many caregivers find that as their role in the relationship changes from being a lover and partner to being primarily a caregiver, the desire for sex with their husband or wife also changes.

This may be confusing for the person with dementia and may cause discord between you both, and frustration and confusion for the person with dementia. This requires gentle conversation, which may need to take place several times for an adjustment to be made. It may need to be repeated many times. A clear boundary with consistency is needed so you can gradually modify the person's expectations.

There is a need for *consent*, regardless of a diagnosis of dementia. Consent to engage in sex will be indicated by behavioural signs of well-being; for example, the person shows pleasure or willingness to engage with you in sex by continuing to be willing as the sex proceeds. If these signs change and the person becomes withdrawn or distressed or passive, the sex should stop.

Incontinence can also be a problem in relation to sex. Once the person with dementia becomes incontinent it often leads to changes in sexual desire in the caregiving partner. Be patient with yourself and clear about what you want for yourself.

Sex is a way we express love and experience pleasure with the person we love most in the world. When that changes, we need to include other ways to express love. This can be a moment for making sure you use non-verbal signals of love such as holding hands, hugging, smiling, kissing, stroking and generally being warm to each other.

Sexual assault

See also *Trauma*

Many people live with memories of sexual assault in their past. This can leave memories associated with the assault and anxiety to the present day. People with dementia may tend to confuse these memories of past events with present-day experience. Current activities such as undressing, showering or bathing with someone else in the bathroom while they are naked can cause significant anxiety and resistance to engaging in these activities.

In caregiving, be mindful of the risk of retraumatizing a person with dementia by activating such memories and anxieties. Go slowly, use a gentle tone, smile, reassure and stop if the person becomes too activated by the experience. Ensure that they remain covered as much as possible throughout if nakedness is too difficult for them. If they do not want you to touch their genitals or other body areas for washing, give them a cloth and ask them to do it themselves.

Sexual disinhibition

See also *Sexual assault*

Sexual disinhibition may be an expression of an unmet need that may communicate a freedom from the usual sexual prohibitions we have and a desire to connect with a partner in a new or enjoyable way.

Sexual disinhibition may also occur in a place or situation that is not socially acceptable. This can be a problem particularly in fronto-temporal dementia, in which the frontal lobes in the brain are significantly affected. This also generally occurs at an earlier age than it does in Alzheimer's and vascular dementia. This form of disinhibition may consist of inappropriate comments, touching or more intrusive actions that constitute sexual assault. This can be traumatizing for others and perhaps for yourself.

If the person with dementia is engaging in this behaviour, it will be necessary to consider the possible meanings of this behaviour and the context in which it occurs. Your response will depend on the meaning of it and the context and likely effect on others. It may mean that you engage with the person or it may mean that you assist them to be more socially appropriate in their expression of their sexuality with others or in public. This may mean that you monitor the person closely when they are in company and are vigilant and ready to prevent it. Or it may mean you consult your GP to explore medical treatments. This is often not desirable but it may be necessary if no other solutions are effective or the situations require more than your vigilance.

Shopping

Trips out to large shopping centres or local shops can be an important stimulus for an enjoyable time together. They can provide much needed interaction with others for the person with dementia and for you. They can also be very stressful for you both if not managed, planned and adapted to the person's needs and capacities.

Preparation for the shopping trip can be an activity in itself. This can involve discussing what you need to buy, which shops you want to visit, searching the fridge or pantry for items you need to purchase, and making a list together. Dressing for the weather is also an important part of planning. You can talk about it while in the bathroom or over breakfast. However, if the person is prone to becoming anxious, it may be best to avoid this preparation and leave it to the last minute to tell them what is to happen or invite them to go shopping.

Shopping centres involve high levels of stimulation with noise, visual activity and smells. You may want to think about what the person can manage and adjust your timing of the trip out so that there is minimal activity around them, such as going early in the morning.

Short-term memory

See also *Long-term memory*, *Memory*

Much has already been written in this book about memory. However, short-term memory (STM) is such a vital part of our memory function and it is so deeply affected in dementia that it deserves particular attention.

This form of memory is often termed 'working memory', as it is the type of memory we use from moment to moment to work with pieces of information, some of which we may not need beyond the moment and therefore don't need to store in long-term memory. STM is like the open document on your desktop. Although the brain is not a computer, the analogy works.

Examples of STM use include holding a phone number you can type into your phone and so don't need to remember. It may be an address you need for a few minutes until you get there. Or it may be that you cleaned your teeth this morning or what you had for breakfast. You don't need to hold that in memory longer than the event or in response to the question, 'What did you have for breakfast?'

Short-term memory capacity decreases and is lost more quickly than long-term memory in dementia. So it affects our ability to recall things like what we were just talking about, or why you went into a room. Mind you, I am plagued by that problem and I don't have dementia. The number of times I have had to retrace my steps to remember what I was looking for...

You can support the person with dementia whose STM fails them in a conversation by including the topic repeatedly as the conversation continues. 'As I was just telling John, we're talking about the game on Saturday.' This can be enough to keep the person oriented to the topic and feeling like contributing successfully.

You can support their STM by repetition of the topic or the activity by giving reminders during the day of the reason for the current activity or the purpose of the car journey, or why they are getting dressed to go out.

Shouting

See *Screaming, Yelling*

Sleep

Most of us sleep for about 30 per cent of our lives. Sleep can be disturbed during dementia due to disruption of the brain, particularly the neurotransmitters such as melatonin that help to regulate the sleep-wake cycle.

Sleep is caused by mechanisms in the brain and by external factors such as what we do before sleep, what we drink and what we do in bed or in the bedroom before sleep. So multiple factors need to be considered.

Maintaining a regular routine around sleep is important to help a person with dementia to sleep well. Switch off screens, turn off lights, change into nightwear, brush teeth, talk quietly. Avoid watching TV in bed. Maintain bed for sleep and sex. Ensure that the person gets some exposure to strong light as this helps orient the person to day and night and causes the production of melatonin.

The daytime routine can also affect sleep. This may include getting enough exercise and eating well. Avoid caffeine after 3pm, and sugary drinks after dinner.

If the sleep-wake cycle is disrupted and the person is awake at night and sleeps during the day, you can gradually shift it back to night-day by steadily increasing the time the person is awake during the day.

If the person wakes repeatedly during the night believing it is daytime, you may need to open the curtains to let them see it is dark outside and it is time for sleep. You can also try a warm drink to ready them for sleep again. At least one study has found that magnesium can help people go to sleep quicker and stay asleep longer. Melatonin may also be helpful.

Smell

Smell is one of the five senses and is a cause for appetite. You can use the smell of food to stimulate the person to eat, to come to the table, and to enjoy the food prepared. It is also a stimulus for memory. Past smells that were significant can activate the person to remember the people, the place and the events that they associate with that smell. Lavender, rose or other herbal aromas can be associated with smells of grandparents' cupboards, wardrobes or drawers.

Smiling

The non-verbal act of smiling can be crucial to shift a mood or quell a reaction that might otherwise escalate into a problem. Smile as part of your communication during the activities of daily living and try to ensure that you make eye-contact or at least let the person know from your tone that you feel positive and warm towards them and you will avoid aggression in close personal caregiving.

Socializing

You are made to be in relationship with people. Your relationships help build your identity as a person. Socializing is important for the person with dementia and for you as a caregiver. They need it to sustain their sense of self, their confidence, their verbal skills and their mood. The same applies to you. If you do not socialize beyond your interactions with the person you care for, you may find yourself burned out. You need to recharge the batteries, and socializing with friends or extended family may be important for you. Debriefing is an important part of socializing when you are a caregiver. It may be with one particular friend with whom you feel comfortable and trust. Sometimes just knowing that someone else understands you can make all the difference.

Soiling

See also *Continence*

Soiling can be associated with not recognizing the muscle activity of the bowel as a signal to go to the toilet.

The person with dementia may soil themselves without noticing it. If this occurs in public, ensure that you have a change of underwear for them, take them to a nearby toilet and clean them up with a minimum of fuss. Do not become negative or chastising. Chat about something else while you clean the person. Treat it as a mundane event. Then return to the social setting or ready yourself to go home.

If it occurs at home, it may be in bed, in which case you will need to change sheets in the middle of the night and then return to sleep if possible. Again, treat it as a mundane event without chastising the person.

In order to avoid such events as much as you can, ensure that the person is invited to move their bowels at regular times, perhaps after each meal. Make sure that they have a diet that promotes solid stools, rather than loose stools over which they may have less control. Preparation for a shopping trip may involve an invitation to sit on the toilet prior to leaving the house.

Spirituality

See also *Religion, Faith, Worship*

It may be that the person maintains an interest in their spiritual practices or rituals long into the progress of dementia. You can support this by being aware of the importance of familiar activities for them in maintaining their sense of self. They will likely experience well-being by engaging in practices or handling objects that mean something to them long past the time when they can find words to explain why they are important. Examples include rosary beads, a yarmulke or misbaha, which can be a comfort to people who have previously worn or prayed with them.

Spitting

This is a socially undesirable practice across cultures. However, in some cultures it is tolerated in public. In western cultures it is not tolerated. If the person with dementia engages in spitting, you may need to place receptacles around the house and encourage or train them to use these in preference to spitting anywhere they please. You can also assist them to learn to do it outside if possible.

Stigma

This is treating the person with dementia as an 'other' or different object that is worthy only of criticism. Stigma is felt by many people in society when they are judged by others as different or lacking in some quality to be 'normal'.

Stigma can be alienating and makes people feel like an outsider, as if they do not belong. As a caregiver, you will notice it more clearly than you have in the past. You can avoid it yourself by ensuring that the tone and content of your speech treats the person you care for with equality. Avoid talking to them as if they are children.

Stimulation

This is vital for human functioning. Without it you become bored, shrivel up and die. Stimulation makes brain cells work to make new connections. This makes them more resistant to the effects of the diseases that cause dementia. Stimulation also makes you feel good. It can remind you of yourself.

Stress

A definition of stress is 'a state of worry or mental tension caused by a difficult situation' (World Health Organization, 2023). It is a natural response that alerts you to a risk or threat. Everyone experiences it.

People with dementia can become more stressed than they usually would because their brain does not function in the automatic and smooth way it once did as the various diseases that cause dementia progress. This stress causes activation of the psychological attachment reaction of seeking out someone stronger and wiser who can relieve their stress and help them feel safe and secure again. Often just knowing another person is in the house can be enough to calm the person with dementia.

As a caregiver, you will need to identify the signs of stress in the person with dementia. Stress may show itself in 'disturbed behaviour' or behavioural and psychological symptoms of dementia (BPSD). These are the traditional terms for behaviour that is observed in people with dementia. However, if you take a holistic view of the behaviour as we did in Part I of this book, you can see that most of this behaviour can be understood as signals of distress. It is a form of communication of distress. Why does a person communicate distress? Why not just deal with it themselves? The answer is in our nature. Our early life experiences are of being soothed, comforted and fed by someone who is able to relieve our distress. This early *attachment* relationship sets the tone for later attachments and becomes a template that we utilize in stressful moments later in life. We also use it as a template to form long-term relationships.

Suffering

People with dementia are frequently referred to as 'sufferers', particularly in the media. However, most people with dementia do not suffer, in the sense of enduring unreasonable pain. They may have moments of discomfort and upset but not suffering. If people with dementia experience the well-being they are capable of, they do not experience any more suffering than you and me who do not have dementia.

Suffering for people with dementia can occur if they are not treated with respect and gentle care. It can occur when they are misunderstood and ignored. Any of the negative behaviours identified by Tom Kitwood (1997) can cause suffering of a physical or emotional kind.

As a caregiver, if you have an eye on the well-being of the person you care for, you will ensure that they do not suffer.

Sundowning

Sundowning is the increased distress and *agitation* that commonly occurs in the late afternoon and early evening – as the sun goes down. It is caused by a tired brain, depleted of resources. Simply being awake and functioning is enough to make a person with dementia tired and unable to function well. That includes being able to manage themselves and regulate their own emotions and needs. Some with advanced dementia may exhibit signs of sundowning as soon as they get up in the morning.

It is a human phenomenon that affects us all. Whenever you go over threshold for what you can deal with you become emotional and restless, have difficulty thinking straight and difficulty remembering events and details. This affects three-year-olds and 83-year-olds. It is a function of the brain that you need rest and nourishment in order to perform at your best.

When you see agitation and restlessness all your caregiving should be designed to keep the person under threshold. Over threshold is agitation, restlessness and decreased cognitive function and dysregulated feeling.

A better name for sundowning is 'over-threshold syndrome'. How to treat it? Prevention is better than cure. Ensure that the person is able to rest through the day between periods of activity. As the afternoon lengthens, move into quiet, less stimulating activity. Quieten the home, simplify the demands on the person. Play music they like but be ready to stop if it seems to be too much to process.

Some sensory stimulation can be soothing and enjoyable. This can include aromatherapy, or massage, or a quiet sing-along. Keep it simple and undemanding. Familiar activity is less demanding on the brain. As brain resources are low, reminiscence may be helpful. You may offer to go through a life-story book of photos and narrative with them, simply showing the photographs and telling them their life or family story.

If they become agitated and cannot sit still for long, you might offer them some finger-food to eat and something to drink while they walk. Food and drink usually have a settling effect. Walk quietly with them and carry the finger-food on a plate, if they let you. If not, tell them you will wait for them. If they are looking for family

LIVING WITH A PERSON WITH DEMENTIA

members you can talk about them as you walk. Eventually you might empathize about feeling tired and suggest sitting down for a rest.

Surviving as a carer – Tom Valenta's Ten Golden Hints (Valenta, 2007)

1. Get organized from day one.

2. Don't accept second-rate medical advice.

3. Acquire survival skills – quickly.

4. Accept genuine offers of help.

5. Know when you need respite.

6. Look after yourself.

7. Don't become isolated.

8. Try to make the system work for you.

9. Have a view of the future without making specific plans.

10. Never lose touch with reality.

Swearing

You may find that the person with dementia develops a liking for swearing. Some people like swearing and may have always sworn. If this is the case it may be up to those around them to adjust to the preferences of the person with dementia. They are being consistent with who they have always been. Even if they are adopting new behaviour by swearing it may be up to others to consider adjusting to the change rather than expecting the person with dementia to display some control they do not have.

Sometimes it can be embarrassing if it is done in public or with people who are not used to them doing this. It occurs because of a reduced awareness of social rules or expectations that usually guide and shape our behaviour. It can be a phase the person goes through which will pass as they move to other ways of expressing themselves or lose memory for the words.

You can use a simple rule-learning approach which is detailed below. The simplest approach is to ignore it if possible. However, if the words are particularly offensive to you or others, you may need to teach the person not to say the word(s) by using frequent repetition of a simple rule such as 'I must not swear'. It sounds overly simple but it works if the rule is kept brief and repeated frequently. Frequently means within the span of the person's memory. Several times an hour perhaps. Once you have repeated it frequently you can check if it has been retained by asking the person, 'What is the rule I asked you to repeat?' Notice I avoided the word 'swearing'. We want the person to focus on the rule, not the swearing.

As I said, the simplest approach may be to not make an issue of it but to support the person's expression of themselves by engaging in conversation in a way that enables them to participate as an equal in social life for as long as they are able, and adjusting your support to the level of effort they need.

Talking books and podcasts

If the person can no longer read, they may utilize talking books, audio books and podcasts. The only difficulty may be reduced attention span. If the person reading the book has a calming voice you may simply have it on in the background as you would with music. Podcasts can be useful as they can be focused on the interests of the person. You may have to set it up, but these can provide a means of engaging the person with dementia in satisfying quiet time.

Taste

Taste is one of the five major senses and is a source of pleasure and enjoyment for us all. It is often associated with smell: 'It smelled so beautiful I could almost taste it.' Food tastes and smells go together. As an activity, you can do a taste guessing game by presenting the person with various unnamed flavours to guess the food. You can combine this with smells. Vary food if you can so that it remains interesting and stimulates appetite. With the availability of ready-made meals, it can be easier than you having to prepare meals from scratch. However, ensure that smells of food are available to stimulate appetite and enjoyment.

Teamwork

Dementia caregiving is a team activity. You cannot do it on your own. You cannot and should not isolate yourself. Engage with the local supports, respite teams, home care teams and specialists from the Alzheimer's organization in your country or region to access their information and services. Many have problem-solving hotlines that can help you get through difficult times. Knowing you are not alone, that help is at hand, is a vital way to remain afloat in rough seas.

Tears

See also *Stress, Love, affection*

You may find yourself crying from time to time. Tears are not a sign of weakness or failure. It may be from sadness or it may be stress. Some people cry when they are angry. However, tears are often from feeling overwhelmed (by the anger or other experience) and unable to know what to do with a difficult situation. Perhaps it is also grief about the loss of your life together and the changes in the person you love.

Whatever the reason, crying can be therapeutic. You can feel relieved afterward. You may feel embarrassed crying in front of others, but this can be healthy if they now know exactly how much distress you are feeling and that you need their support.

Teeth

Dental hygiene is important when you have dementia. It can be difficult, however, to get the person with dementia to brush their teeth. This can create a problem with tooth decay if long periods pass without teeth being cleaned.

Tooth decay can cause pain that can go undetected because the behaviour it causes looks like distress behaviour rather than pain behaviour. When decayed teeth are removed the behavioural issue can resolve. This is not an argument for removing teeth. On the contrary, it is to emphasize the importance of dental care and of looking at all possible causes of behavioural disturbance.

Dental care should be regular and part of the morning and

nightly routine to ensure it is accepted and maintained. To help the person become accustomed to you supporting them to brush their teeth you can engage in 'show me your teeth' in a smile and introduce a pleasant tasting toothpaste. Make your instructions simple and direct. Smile. Open wide. Comment on what you are doing and praise on completion. 'What beautiful teeth you have. What a lovely smile you have.'

However, it is not always necessary to have the person open their mouth wide and have you do the teeth cleaning for them. I am grateful to Jackie Pool for the following insight from her experience as an occupational therapist and dementia care practitioner for many years. It may be better to support the person with dementia with the hand-under-hand technique in which you offer your hand under theirs. They hold the brush and you move your hand with their hand resting on yours so they are free to move, with you supportively stimulating the action without taking over. That way the act of teeth-cleaning is a partnership that can be completed without distress but with a sense of accomplishment.

Telling lies

A person with dementia is no more likely to tell lies than anyone else. We all do it from time to time, depending on the reason and the importance of it. The most likely reason for a person with dementia to tell lies is to cover their mistakes or their inability to do something, to preserve self-esteem and avoid shame. It can also be due to feeling cornered by questioning. This is the motive behind most children's lies.

So, if the person makes a mistake, do not blame them or react with disappointment or anger. Accept it without making much of it. Your non-verbal acceptance of the mistake will be important here because they will have a radar for detecting criticism. Don't go on about how acceptable it is to make mistakes. This just emphasizes the fact they made a mistake. Just move on.

It may be that the person is confabulating. This is telling a story that is based on memory or fantasy rather than fact in order to make sense of the current situation. It is not intentionally lying in order to deceive. It may also be an attempt to be socially competent by engaging in storytelling as everyone else does.

Temperature

The person with dementia may not be able to adjust their behaviour to the temperature or be aware that the temperature is too hot or cold for comfort. This can cause them to over- or under-dress for the occasion. It can also cause hypothermia or over-heating and dehydration. This latter issue can be a problem if the person walks a lot and refuses to stop for meals or drinks. What is a warm day to you can be a real problem for a person who cannot adjust their dress or behaviour to the conditions.

As a caregiver, you will need to monitor their clothing for over- or under-dressing and check their hydration by increasing frequency of drinks. If they do not take water regularly (and many older people prefer tea or coffee, both of which have a diuretic effect), they may benefit from a frozen confectionery made from electrolyte solution. Offering a cold compress for their face can also help maintain a good temperature. And monitor the temperature of the house so they have access to cool or warm spaces as the case may be.

If the person becomes heat-stressed, cool them quickly with a cold compress on the forehead and place their forearms in cold water. Seek medical advice if they do not improve.

Time-out for you

Take time out for yourself as a caregiver. It is an important part of self-care to have relief with some part of your day or week in which you switch off from caregiving. This may mean you have to organize someone to come and stay with the person you care for until you return. Respite is part of time-out for you. Organize it and plan ahead so you have a break to look forward to and support ready at hand.

Tiredness

Read your own signs of tiredness. These may be difficulty staying awake, irritability, headaches, aches and pains, difficulty making decisions, anxiety and moodiness. If you deal with your tiredness regularly, you will remain an active and effective caregiver. If you

A–Z OF DEMENTIA CARE AT HOME

do not, and you ignore the signs of tiredness, you may burn out rather quickly. You cannot maintain a cracking pace for a long time. None of us can.

Ask others for help. Take advantage of times a paid caregiver comes to help with personal care and go for a coffee or a walk. Arrange a regular meetup with a friend. Tell someone about your tiredness, do not keep it to yourself. Exercise, socialize and eat well. Remember the four pillars of a healthy life.

Toilet

See also *Hygiene, Privacy, Dressing, Continence*

Going to the toilet is a complex activity that requires the coordination of many brain parts to be successful. So in dementia, it can easily go wrong.

First is the awareness that the person needs to urinate or defecate. This requires an awareness of the sensation in the muscles of a full bladder or bowel. In dementia, this can be difficult for the person to recognize, resulting in failing to make it in time or not at all.

If the person does make it in time, they have to then successfully remove clothing. They may need your help to do this. The quicker and simpler you can do this the better. Keep your efforts to a minimum so they do not become flustered and anxious, and lose focus on what they are there for.

It is helpful if you can get males to sit on the toilet for urinating as well as defecating. This prevents accidental spilling of urine outside the toilet bowl. Do not hurry them off the toilet. Give them time to empty their bladder or bowel. For males and females, a bladder can be slow to empty. Give it time. After they have finished defecating, wait until the person has urinated. Usually when a person defecates, the end of the process is signalled by urinating as muscles return to normal. If the person is tempted to hurry off the toilet, you may decide to read them a story from the newspaper or a book so they sit still for a while longer.

Cleaning the person may be your job as well if they are not reliable at it or unable to do it. You will get used to doing it. Keep it simple and matter-of-fact. Do not go on about it. If you are male

205

and not used to doing this for your wife or female partner, you will need to know that you wipe from the front toward the back so faeces do not contact the vagina.

Re-dress the person and check that they are fully clothed and ready to leave the toilet. Ensure hygiene by washing hands thoroughly with soap and water as part of the post-toilet routine.

Tone of voice

See also *Communication, Non-verbal communication*

Your tone of voice communicates your mood and intention. It is a vital part of your non-verbal communication. When people with dementia cannot make sense of verbal communication as readily as they once did, non-verbal communication channels take on greater importance. Avoid the sing-song tone and pitch of an adult speaking to a child. Listen for it in yourself. If you pick it up, try to speak normally in a conversational tone.

Touch

This is one of the five major senses, or channels of information to the brain. Touch can give us pleasure and comfort. When we are comfortable and wearing clothes that fit, being touched by a person we love and who loves us, we feel good and experience pleasure and joy. Pleasurable touch is important for the well-being of people with dementia. It may be holding hands, or stroking the person's face or arms or hands.

Some people are not comfortable with a lot of touch and will become agitated and anxious if you touch them. Always check it out to see what effect your touch is having. If the person is your long-term partner you will already know this, but bear in mind that preferences can change in the context of dementia. Keep updating what you do in the light of how the person is currently acting.

Trauma

See also *Abuse, Assault, Privacy, Sexual assault* and *Post-traumatic stress disorder*

Trauma is not in the event, but in the person who experiences the event. Two people can be robbed but only one becomes traumatized. Personality style, previous trauma history, having other mental health problems, no or few family or other social supports, or a history of substance abuse can all contribute to an event becoming traumatic.

Not everyone who becomes traumatized develops PTSD. About 15 per cent of people exposed to traumatic events will develop PTSD.

Regardless of whether a person has a diagnosis of PTSD you may notice that the person acts anxiously or is irritated and reactive in certain situations. This can indicate that the person is having a traumatic reaction and finds the activity traumatizing. It may be as simple as having you remaining in the bathroom while they remove their clothes to urinate or to prepare for a shower or bath. Removing clothing can be an occasion for anxious activation of past traumas.

As the person loses memories and is unable to make sense of everyday activities as reliably as they once did, they can be more prone to anxious traumatic reactions. This is discussed in detail in *Post-traumatic stress disorder*.

Treachery

Tom Kitwood (1997) defines treachery as 'using forms of deception in order to distract or manipulate a person, or force them into compliance' (p.46). This act may be well motivated but usually diminishes you and them. For example, 'Your husband will be back soon', when you know they will not as they died some years ago. There are many approaches to this issue. Some say it's okay to deceive the person with dementia if it prevents them being distressed. Others say it is a betrayal of them as it uses their memory problems and difficulty understanding against them. Others say it fails to explore whether they might be capable of adjusting if they had this information repeated every time they wanted to have their husband with them.

A culture of deception as a legitimate way to treat people with dementia has become accepted in many western countries, often by professionals who work in this area of healthcare. In this deception culture, it is okay to tell white lies, to collude with false stories in a family, to use tricks to pretend the buses do not run today or you have lost your keys and cannot go to the shops, going along with the erroneous information that their husband will be returning soon.

All of these forms of treachery sell the person short and sell you short as a caregiver. There are other ways to respond that can explore what capacities the person and you have to work through these situations.

First, find out what the person's need is in the situation. Looking for a husband is likely to be an *attachment* need. If so, empathize with that need and engage in a conversation with them about their husband. The fact that he has died may come up. In some part of her she will likely know he has died and the grief of this can come up along with the loving feelings, and the pain of loss can be comforted. Tomorrow she may return to this desire for him and the conversation about him can occur again. Each time it is addressed, his death will become more memorable to the point where she may only need a gentle reminder that he has died and will then return to her afternoon.

Trust

Trust is crucial in dementia care. Trust in any relationship is built on being reliable and predictable. This is critical for the person with dementia to be able to function in an unpredictable world that they have difficulty making sense of. You can become a safe harbour of security for them if you are reliable and treat them with respect and gentle kindness. People with dementia are capable of experiencing hopeful and enjoyable lives if the care environment is safe and secure, stimulating, forgiving and pleasurable.

Unsafe leaving

Unsafe leaving refers to the fact that sometimes a person with dementia may leave where they are in a manner that is unsafe, seeking another place, usually a place they think of as home. Or they may be seeking stimulation. This is a term often used in long-term care to describe someone leaving without permission or against the wishes of the management.

It can cause a safety concern for the person with dementia as they may or may not have an awareness of the need to prepare to travel with adequate money, clothing appropriate to the weather conditions, and food and drink for the journey. They may also not have a clear idea of where to go or how to get where they want to go, be safe around traffic, or know how to return.

Because of memory loss and lack of a clear idea of the route to their destination they can become easily disoriented, confused and eventually lost.

The desire for home is deep in us. If the person with dementia is wanting to be in another place, it may be that they want to visit a particular house that was once home. The attachment to a home is a feeling that is activated by memories of past people, activities, animals and objects. An attachment is a connection to any of these. It may be that they want to go home to their mother because of a sense that they have to be home by dark. This can become a strong motivator as the day ends and the person feels the need to finish what they are doing and go home to their parents, usually mother. This may occur at night when the person gets an urge to return to home. You may have to get in the car together and drive until they are more peaceful and ready to return to their current home with you. On the journey you may find it helpful to talk about their early life. You may ask questions about their mother, what they used to do and what she was like.

Some have suggested that tracking technology is important to use so that the person with dementia can be located quickly and easily. In recent years it has become less obtrusive and easily worn. There remain ethical concerns about restriction of freedom of movement and intrusion on privacy that have been discussed widely and will continue to be discussed. However, this type of technology in the form of a smart watch or similar has begun to be more widely accepted. It is used more by parents to track the movement of children and has become more accepted among carers of people living with dementia.

Urinary tract infections (UTIs)

UTIs cause significant distress for people with dementia, female and male. They usually become delirious with confusion, agitation, fluctuating awareness and cognitive ability, and significant discomfort. On top of their dementia difficulties, the person's ability to function with a UTI can be drastically reduced.

Treatment is antibiotics. The sooner you can get this treatment for the person the better. An infection like a UTI can often be like a comet with a sudden onset and a long tail of symptoms that can last weeks after the infection has been treated.

Validation

Validation is the acceptance and understanding of the perspective and experience of the person with dementia and responding to it at the level of feeling. It is accepting the subjective truth of the perspective for the person without challenge or question. It is effectively saying, 'I believe this is what it is like for you', 'I can see this upset you deeply', even though the person may be hallucinating or delusional.

Responding with empathy is an important ingredient of a validating response. It may mean responding to a person who is delusional about their mother still being alive in the following way:

Caregiver: So you are on your way to see your mother? What is she normally doing at this time of the day?

Diane: She'll be picking up the kids from school. She always walked us home.

Caregiver: What did you do when you got home?

Diane: We had a glass of milk and a biscuit. Then we went outside to play until tea time. Mum cooked tea.

Caregiver: What was your mum like when you were a child?

Diane: She was pretty.

This dialogue gives you an idea of the tone that validation takes. You start from their perspective. Avoid the question 'Why?' as that can be experienced as a challenge to explain and justify their belief that their mother is at home and alive.

Being understood with validation is often calming and enables you to establish a connection of trust and understanding when the person may be needing attachment – which is likely the reason the desire to visit mother has emerged.

Vascular dementia

This type of dementia is caused by repeated small strokes that affect the person usually in a stepwise manner. However, vascular ageing can be progressive and causes gradual decline in the health of blood vessels that supply the brain. Losses of function depend on the location of the stroke. This is very different from Alzheimer's dementia, which usually has a generally predictable progress.

For more information on this and other common causes of dementia, explore your local Alzheimer's Association website.

VIPS

This is a model of person-centred care and an approach to guide care, created by Professor Dawn Brooker using the acronym for Very Important Persons to describe person-centred care. The four elements are Value, Individual, Perspective and Social. For more on this see *Person-centred care.*

Value: The person has intrinsic worth regardless of their personal characteristics or disabilities. They are respected for who they are.

Individual: Care is provided to the person according to their individual needs rather than a one-size-fits-all approach commonly seen in traditional dementia care. Individual life stories and personal characteristics are important ways of connecting to the person.

Perspective: The point-of-view of the person with dementia is protected and sustained in care interactions. The caregiver adjusts to the perspective and dispositions of the person and makes them a priority.

Social: We are social beings who need relationships and have been formed in relationships throughout our lives. Care must respect this need by valuing the social connections of the person and sustaining their capacity to relate with others through language, both verbal and non-verbal.

Vision

This is one of the five major sensory channels through which you engage with the world around you. This is important for people with dementia, as, along with hearing, it is a major source of information about the world.

Some people with dementia may have had a vision impairment all their lives and now have a cognitive impairment as well. In this situation, it may be important to support their well-learned strategies for coping with a visually impaired world and ensure that they have other sensory cues to support their mobility and use of the physical world. Socially, appropriately clear language may be crucial to providing them with cues to negotiate the world.

Others with dementia may develop a visual impairment. If this is the case, your role as carer may be to simplify the physical environment, use clear visual cues and improve way-finding and walking surfaces. Keep the home as familiar as possible. However, if necessary, remove objects that can be a problem for bumping into or knocking over. Ensure that the person can use objects such as utensils and crockery. It may be necessary to obtain modified utensils. These are readily available through services that support people with disabilities and other impairments.

Use colour and symbols or signs to assist way-finding. If finding the toilet is a problem, paint the door a bright colour or attach a drawing of a familiar type of toilet on it so they can find it easily and quickly. 'If you need the toilet, look for the blue door.' It may be that reading the word 'toilet' is no longer possible, in which case the drawing of the object they are looking for can be useful. It can also help to have enlarged images or text.

Modifying the kitchen can also help. This applies also to the cupboard and drawers. Perhaps take cupboard doors off so the person can see the objects they are looking for without having to search or replace the objects in the wrong location. Label drawer compartments but be patient when this does not work effectively.

There is a great deal known about the ideal physical environment for people with dementia. Make use of this knowledge either online or by engaging your local Alzheimer's Association support.

Visiting

Visits to home are an important way to maintain social connection and the skills for interaction with others. Visits by family sustain the sense of belonging and inclusion.

You may need to educate family members and friends to introduce themselves by name so the person with dementia can recognize them and activate old memories. Have a photograph album or other stimulus ready (or ask the visitor to bring something along with them) to use during the visit so the person with dementia can be engaged in something that activates shared memories.

Perhaps sing together if that is a shared activity they may enjoy, or make something together in a structured way that includes everyone or gives you, the caregiver, a rest for a few minutes. This requires a bit of preparation but can be very effective. It also helps the visitor by giving them something to do while they visit. The shared activity can become enjoyable and memorable.

Vocabulary

The range of words a person with dementia is able to use will change over time, gradually reducing. This is especially true for Alzheimer's dementia, which is characterized by word-finding difficulty in the early stages (particularly nouns), followed by loss of sentence structure. As a caregiver you can support the person with words that you know they are looking for. Wait a heart-beat before you provide it so they can search for it and then offer the word you think they are looking for.

Wandering

This is a term used to describe what people with dementia do when they walk. It is often used in a negative way to mean walking without purpose. Nothing could be further from the truth. There is always a reason and a purpose.

It may be that the person walks because they are searching for someone, or they are bored and looking for something to do. It may be that they walk to exercise.

It always has a purpose. Avoid the term 'wandering'; use 'walking' instead.

War

Wartime memories and experience may come to mind for veterans who have dementia. They may have been able to manage these memories without too much intrusion into their lives. However, with the onset of dementia they may lose some of the ability to keep the memories at bay. This can cause distress to them and to those closest to them. As a caregiver, you may find you become caught up in the memories or mistaken for enemy combatants and become a focus for aggression. If this occurs, you must act to protect yourself. Speak about it to someone you trust, preferably a GP who can help you with connections for support or with medication that can soothe the person's agitation and anxiety.

Some ex-prisoners of war may become delusional if they lose body weight to a weight they were during their captivity. They can experience dependency as being like their captivity. They may mistake you for a captor. This can be distressing for you both.

Way-finding

In your home you may benefit from having written signs or pictures of objects that you want the person to find, such as a toilet. Place this sign or picture on the toilet door. Make sure the picture looks like the toilet they are familiar with. If the person with dementia fails to recognize objects from current life but does recognize objects from younger years, use a picture of a toilet they will recognize. Way-finding can also be improved by painting the toilet door a vivid colour and teaching the person to associate the coloured door with 'toilet'.

Use night-lights to assist night activity so they can find the toilet or kitchen and so on easily and quickly.

In the kitchen, you might consider taking cupboard doors off and replacing them with clear glass or Perspex doors so the person can locate objects that are kept in cupboards. Drawers can be labelled but this depends on ability to recognize written language.

Well-being

Well-being is a subjective state in which a person experiences pleasure, satisfaction, contentment. Signs of well-being and ill-being have been identified by Tom Kitwood (1997) and are listed in the Appendix.

Will

If the person with dementia is your spouse or partner, you should both have a will in place as soon as possible so that in the event of either of you dying your estate and affairs can be taken care of. Know where it is and who is the executor.

Withdrawal

Withdrawal usually occurs if a person is depressed or has lost confidence in their ability to function with others. Depression is more common in dementia and may need to be treated with medication. However, the initial response to noticing social withdrawal should be a social one. This should improve the frequency or type of social interactions, and the person with dementia should be monitored for any specific reason that may be causing the withdrawal. It may be that the person needs more scaffolding of social interactions so it is easier to be successful and they do not experience so much frustration or failure.

Work

Occupation is one of the five fundamental needs. If the person with dementia can continue their work, they should be encouraged to do so for as long as possible. There may be ways they can still be productive and engaged that are discreetly supported so they continue to experience success and a sense of efficacy.

Worship

See also *Church*, *Faith*, *Spirituality*

This has been discussed under several headings. The ritual and routine of worship can be soothing and provide a way to be among others that is highly supported and positive without huge demands for individual contribution.

Writing

Writing may gradually deteriorate as dementia progresses, not only because of word-finding difficulty but because the fine motor control required for writing may be impaired. The person may gradually lose the ability to hold a pen but may be able to hold a paintbrush or other writing implement. It may be possible to modify and support writing by making changes to how it is achieved.

Yelling

See also *Screaming*

Yelling is an indication of distress. Ask yourself what might be causing it. Check for physical sources of pain or discomfort. Then check for emotional causes of distress. This will enable you to find a cause and modify it. Medication may be useful but try psychosocial approaches first.

Younger onset dementia

Younger onset dementia occurs in people under 65 years of age. The diseases that cause dementia in younger people are similar to those that cause it in older people. However, there are several differences that make the onset of dementia in younger people particularly difficult for them and for those living with them.

At a younger age, dementia can occur when the person has children at home, and when they have financial commitments and a developing career. There is often a partner in mid-career who faces the reality of leaving their career and becoming a carer. A husband or wife can gradually lose their role as partner and can become a carer for their spouse. Teenage and younger children can lose the parent they had and have to come to grips with a parent whose personality is changing. This can make parenting difficult for the other parent and hard for the children, who can struggle to make sense of unpredictable parenting. In short, the disruption can be socially, financially and occupationally significant for the entire young family.

The most prominent problems in younger onset dementia can be caused by changes in executive function. These include the abilities to think, to plan, to organize oneself, to manage one's behaviour in social settings according to social rules of acceptable behaviour, to manage one's emotions, to stop oneself, and to initiate behaviour.

Specifically, sexual behaviour may become difficult if the person cannot control thoughts and urges that are usually appropriate to express between consenting partners in private, but which may not be appropriate in public and when younger people or strangers are involved. Such behaviour can occur if the person with dementia is losing an awareness of socially appropriate behaviour and the ability to manage this behaviour.

As with older onset dementia, younger people with dementia are best served by a person-centred approach that considers their physical health, personality, the neurological condition that is progressing, their social and emotional needs and their personal life story.

There is a lack of support services available in most countries for families who have a member with younger onset dementia. Most dementia support services are shaped for older adults. However, there is an increasing awareness of the need to provide services that address the unique circumstance of families and individuals with younger onset dementia. You may find your local dementia support services are your best port of call to find your way into what is available for you and your family.

Appendix

Signs of well-being

- Communicating wishes/needs successfully
- Engaging with the people, things and events around them
- Sensitive to the emotional needs of others
- Positive mood (e.g. smiling, laughing)
- Engaging in creative activity such as painting, singing, dancing
- Enjoying interactions with others
- Aware of the well-being of others by being helpful
- Initiating conversation with others
- Affectionate
- Self-respecting in attention to dress and appearance
- Physically relaxed (e.g. facial expression and body posture)
- Showing humour, playfulness
- Cooperating with requests
- Making eye contact
- Confident
- Cheerful

APPENDIX

- Willingly participating in care
- Trusting others
- Comfortable with physical closeness (e.g. being touched)

Signs of ill-being

- Negative mood (showing upset in facial expression, posture and sounds, such a whimpering, calling out, screaming or crying)
- Walking into other people's private space or into unsafe areas
- Grieving, sad
- Angry, aggressive
- Agitated or restless
- Showing anxiety or fear
- Boredom
- Bodily tension
- Easily dominated by others
- Being rejected or ignored by others
- Lethargy, slowness, apathy
- Withdrawal
- Physical discomfort or pain
- Unable to enjoy things, flat
- Lonely or socially isolated
- Making noise, calling out or vocalizing
- Verbally refusing care
- Suspicious of others
- Physically threatening others

References

Australian Institute of Health and Welfare (2024). *Dementia in Australia: Web report*. AIHW, Australian Government, accessed 17 November 2024.

Brooker, D. & Latham, I. (2015). *Person-Centred Dementia Care: Making Services Better with the VIPS Framework* (2nd edition). London: Jessica Kingsley Publishers.

Keats, J. (1899). *The Complete Poetical Works and Letters of John Keats*, Cambridge Edition. Boston, MA: Houghton, Mifflin and Company.

Kitwood, T. (1997, 2019). *Dementia Reconsidered: The Person Still Comes First* (second edition). London: Open University Press.

Miesen, B. & Jones, G. (1992). *Caregiving in Dementia: Research and Applications*. London and New York, NY: Routledge.

Post, S.G. (2000). *The Moral Challenge of Alzheimer Disease: Ethical Issues from Diagnosis to Dying* (second edition). Baltimore, MD: Johns Hopkins University Press.

Taylor-Desir, M. (2022). *What is posttraumatic stress disorder (PTSD)?* American Psychiatric Association. www.psychiatry.org/patients-families/ptsd/what-is-ptsd. Accessed 28 October 2024.

Tronick, E. & Gold, C.M. (2020). *The Power of Discord*. London: Little Brown Spark.

Valenta, T. (2007). *Remember Me, Mrs V? Caring for My Wife: Her Alzheimer's and Others' Stories*. Melbourne, Australia: Michelle Anderson Publishing.

World Health Organization (2023). *Package of Interventions for Rehabilitation*. www.who.int/teams/noncommunicable-diseases/sensory-functions-disability-and-rehabilitation/rehabilitation/service-delivery/package-of-interventions-for-rehabilitation. Accessed 23 October 2024.

World Health Organization (2024). *Abuse of older people*. www.who.int/health-topics/abuse-of-older-people. Accessed 24 April 2024.

List of Topics

A

ABC model of behaviour management, 59, 64, 74, 89
Absconding, **53**, 175
Abuse, 53, **54**, 69, 73, 175, 187, 206
Accusations, **55**
Activity, **56**, 78
Adynamia, **57**, 107
Aggression, **57**, 117, 127, 175
Agitation, **60**, 155
Agnosia, **61**
Alcohol, **62**
All-or-nothing thinking, **62**, 77, 85
Alzheimer's disease, **63**, 98
Announcing care, **63**
Annoyed, **63**
Antecedent, **64**
Anti-anxiety medication, **64**, 148
Antidepressant medication, **64**, 100, 148
Antipsychotic medication, **65**, 148, 176
Anxiety, 64, **65**
Apathy, **67**, 135, 163
Art, **67**, 151
Assault, 54, **68**, 73, 131, 175, 187, 206
Assertiveness, **69**
Assisting, **69**, 147
Attachment, **70**, 83, 103, 132, 161, 208
Attention, **70**
Attention-seeking, **70**, 175

B

Back off, **71**

Bathing, **72**, 131
Bedwetting, **74**, 89, 91, 135
Behaviour, **74**
Behaviour Support Team, **75**, 119
Behavioural consequences, **75**
Bereavement, **76**, 187
Black-and-white thinking, 63, **77**
Boredom, **77**
Boundaries, **78**
Brain, **78**
Brain cells, **79**
Burnout, **79**, 122, 185

C

Caregiving, **80**
Catastrophizing, **81**, 85
Causes, behavioural, 75, **81**, 175
Celebration, **81**
Challenging behaviour, **81**, 103, 175
Choices, **82**
Church, **83**, 182, 216
Closeness, **83**
Cognitive behavioural therapy (CBT), **84**
Cognitive distortions, 62, **85**
Cognitive rehabilitation (CR), **85**
Cognitive stimulation therapy (CST), **85**
Collaboration, **86**
Comfort, **86**, 132
Communication, **86**, 206
Competence, legal, **87**
Compliments, praise, **88**
Confabulation, **88**

221

LIVING WITH A PERSON WITH DEMENTIA

Consent, **88**, 191
Consequences, 75, **89**
Continence, 74, **89**, 135, 196, 205
Conversation, **91**
Cooperation, **92**
Coordination problems, **92**
Creativity, **92**
Cynicism, **93**

D

Dad, **93**
Dance, **94**
Death, **94**, 183
Decision-making, **95**
Defences, **96**
Defensiveness, **96**
Delusions, 40, **96**, 123, 176
Delirium, **97**
Dementia, 63, **98**
Denial, 96, **99**, 185
Dentist, **100**
Depression, 77, **100**
Dignity, 73, **100**
Disempowerment, **101**, 147
Disparagement, **101**, 147
Disruption, **102**
Distraction, **102**
Distress behaviour, 35, 82, **102**, 103, 175
Disturbed behaviour, 81, **103**, 175
Domestic tasks, **103**
Double entendre, **104**
Dressing, 61, **104**, 205
Driving, **105**
Dying, **105**

E

Eating, 61, 70, **106**, 115, 147, 159
Emotions, **107**, 117
Empathy, **109**
Empowerment, 101, **110**, 172
End of life, **110**, 161
Enjoyment, **110**
Ethics, **111**
Excess disability, **112**, 134, 175
Executive function, **112**
Exercise, **113**, 126

F

Facilitation, **113**
Faith, 83, **113**, 182, 196, 216
Family, **114**, 183
Fear of strangers, **114**
Fears, **115**
Feeding, 70, **115**
Feelings, **116**
Financial planning, **117**
Finger-food, 47, 107, **117**, 147, 148
Fitness, **119**
Forgetting, **119**, 145, 149
Friends, **120**

G

Gardening, **120**
Gestures, **121**
Going out, **121**
Guardianship, **122**
Guilt, **122**, 185

H

Hallucinations, 96, **123**, 165, 176
Happiness, **125**
Health, **125**
Hearing, **126**
Helplessness, **126**
Hitting, **127**
Hobbies, **128**
Holding, **128**
Home, **128**
Hope, **129**
Housework, **129**
Hugging, **129**, 145
Humour, **130**, 138
Hunger, **130**
Hygiene, 73, **131**, 155, 205

I

Identity, 73, **131**
Ignoring, **132**, 147
Ill-being, **132**
Illness, **133**
Implicit memory, **133**
Imposition, **134**, 147, 154
Inclusion, **134**, 172
Incontinence, 74, 90, 91, **135**, 191
Independence, **135**
Indifference, **135**

LIST OF TOPICS

Infantilization, **136**, 139, 147
Insomnia, **136**
Intact abilities, **137**
Intimacy, **137**
Intimidation, **138**, 147
Invalidation, **138**, 147

J
Jokes, **138**
Joy, **138**

L
Labelling, **139**, 139, 147
Language, **139**
Laughter, **139**
Learning, **140**
Leaving home, **140**
Lewy body dementia (LBD), **140**
Life story, **141**, 183
Light, **142**
Likes/dislikes, **142**
Limit setting, **143**
Listening, active, **143**
Long-term memory, **145**, 149, 193
Love, affection, **145**
Lying, **146**

M
Malignant social psychology, **147**
Mealtimes, 70, **147**, 159
Medication, 64, **148**
Memory, **149**, 193
Mirroring, 107, 110, **149**
Mirrors, **149**
Mistakes, **150**
Misunderstood, being, **150**
Mobility, loss of, **151**
Mocking, **151**
Mother, **151**
Motivation for behaviour, **151**, 175
Music, **152**

N
Nagging, **153**
Nakedness, **153**
Names, **154**
Needs, **154**
Negotiation, 131, **154**
Noise, **155**

Non-verbal communication, **156**, 206

O
Objectification, **157**
Obsessions, **157**
Occupation, 77, **158**
Outbursts, **158**
Outpacing, **159**
Overeating, **159**

P
Pain, 60, **160**
Palliative care, 106, 110, **161**
Parents, **161**
Passivity, 135, **163**
Pauses in conversation, **164**
Perception, **164**
Personality, **166**
Person-centred care, 80, **167**
Personhood, 119, **168**
Photographs, 114, **169**, 183
Physical environment, **169**
Play, **170**
Positioning, **171**
Positive and Negative Signs Scale
    (PANSIS), **172**
Positive person work, **172**
Post-traumatic stress disorder
    (PTSD), **172**, 206
Power battles, **174**
Privacy, 54, 73, 131, **174**, 205, 206
Problem behaviour, 103, **175**
Psychological therapies, 84, **175**
Psychosis, **176**
Punishment, **176**
Purpose, sense of, **177**

Q
Quality of life, **177**

R
Reaching through dementia, **178**
Reactions to behaviour, **178**
Reading, **178**
Reality orientation, **179**
Recall memory, **180**
Recognition memory, **180**
Recognizing faces, **180**
Recreation, **180**

Refusal, **181**
Regression, 96, **181**
Reinforcement, **181**
Relationships, **182**
Relatives, **182**
Religion, 83, **182**, 196
Reminiscence, 114, **183**
Repair, **183**
Repetitiveness, **183**
Repression, 96, **188**
Reprimand, **185**
Respite, 122, **185**
Routine, daily, **186**

S
Sadness, 117, **187**
Safeguarding, 54, **187**
Scaffolding, 47, 113, **187**
Scolding, **187**
Screaming, **188**, 194, 216
Sedation, **188**
Self, **189**
Self-esteem, **189**
Self-harm, **190**
Sex, 137, **190**
Sexual assault, **191**, 192, 206
Sexual disinhibition, **192**
Shopping, **192**
Short-term memory, 145, 149, **193**
Shouting, **194**
Sleep, **194**
Smell, **195**
Smiling, **195**
Socializing, **195**
Soiling, 74, 91, 135, **196**
Spirituality, 83, 182, **196**, 216
Spitting, **197**
Stigma, **197**
Stimulation, 49, **197**
Stress, **197**, 202
Suffering, **198**
Sundowning, 60, **199**
Surviving as a carer – Tom Valenta's Ten Golden Hints, **200**
Swearing, **200**

T
Talking books and podcasts, **201**
Taste, **201**
Teamwork, **202**
Tears, **202**
Teeth, 97, 100, **202**
Telling lies, 88, **203**
Temperature, **204**
Time-out for you, **204**
Tiredness, **204**
Toilet, 73, **205**
Tone of voice, **206**
Touch, **206**
Trauma, 54, 69, 73, 191, **206**
Treachery, **207**
Trust, **208**

U
Unsafe leaving, 53, 140, **208**
Urinary tract infections (UTIs), **209**

V
Validation, 42, 163, 172, **210**
Vascular dementia, **211**
VIPS, **211**
Vision, **212**
Visiting, 62, **213**
Vocabulary, **213**

W
Wandering, 48, 119, **213**
War, **214**
Way-finding, 49, **214**
Well-being, 73, **215**
Will, **215**
Withdrawal, **215**
Work, **215**
Worship, 196, **216**
Writing, **216**

Y
Yelling, 194, **216**
Younger onset dementia, 99, **216**